5:2
YOUR LIFE

5:2

YOUR LIFE

*GET HAPPY,
HEALTHY
AND SLIM*

KATE HARRISON

This edition first published in Great Britain in 2014 by
Orion
an imprint of the Orion Publishing Group Ltd
Orion House, 5 Upper St Martin's Lane,
London WC2H 9EA
An Hachette UK Company

5 7 9 10 8 6

A CIP catalogue record for this book is available
from the British Library.

Mass Market Paperback ISBN: 978 1 4091 5496 9

Printed in Great Britain by CPI Group (UK) Ltd, Croydon CR0 4YY

The Orion Publishing Group's policy is to use papers that are natural, renewable
and recyclable and made from wood grown in sustainable forests. The logging
and manufacturing processes are expected to conform to the environmental
regulations of the country of origin.

Every effort has been made to ensure that the information in the book is
accurate. The information in this book will be relevant to the majority of
people but may not be applicable in each individual case so it is advised that
professional medical advice is obtained for specific health matters. Neither the
publisher nor author accepts any legal responsibility for any personal injury
or other damage or loss arising from the use of the information in this book.
Anyone making a change in their diet should consult their GP especially if
pregnant, infirm, elderly or under 16.

Every effort has been made to fulfil requirements with regard to reproducing
copyright material. The author and publisher will be glad to rectify any
omissions at the earliest opportunity.

www.orionbooks.co.uk

Important health notes

This book is written for information only and is not intended as medical advice, or as a substitute for medical advice, diagnosis or treatment. It includes links for information and interest but the author and publisher have no control over their contents. You should always consult a doctor before making dietary changes or beginning an exercise plan.

Children, teenagers and pregnant and breastfeeding women should not fast.

If you have diabetes, a chronic medical condition, or any history of eating disorders, it's particularly important that you consult your doctor, specialist or diabetes nurse, before embarking on the 5:2 Diet or any diet.

Neither the author nor publisher or associates can be held responsible for any loss or claim resulting from the use or misuse of information and suggestions contained in this book, or for the failure to take medical advice.

Finally, never disregard professional medical advice or delay medical treatment because of something you have read in this book.

Additional support

The 5:2 Life Plan is based on tried and tested, practical exercises to improve your quality of life. However, if you are suffering from depression or any other mental health issues, it's advised that you consult your doctor or specialist about the suitability of the exercises.

In addition, if you are planning to give up smoking, please do take advantage of the advice and support you can gain from your family doctor or surgery. It will improve your chances of success!

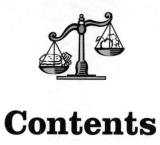

Contents

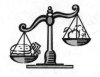

INTRODUCTION

Why you should 5:2 Your Life!

ARE you desperate to change your life but can't find the time to make a start? 5:2 could be what you're looking for . . . by making small changes on just two days a week, you can reap the benefits on the other five – improving your relationships, work life, relaxation, fitness and even your sleep . . .

Most of us know there are things we could change to become happier, or healthier, but we struggle to find the time or energy to get started. We think it's going to be a huge, all or nothing effort.

But it doesn't have to be that way . . .

Take the 5:2 diet. We used to believe that dieting meant restricting ourselves the whole time – and feeling guilty when, inevitably, we gave into temptation. But now hundreds of thousands of people find they can reach a healthy, stable weight by watching the calories on just two days each week.

Now imagine applying the same principle to the rest of our lives – making small changes, just twice a week, that will help you achieve your biggest dreams.

1

That's 5:2 Your Life.

I've lost two stone doing the 5:2 diet – after a lifetime of yoyo dieting – but almost as important is what I've gained: bags more energy, a new enthusiasm for running (before this plan I couldn't run for the bus) and the sense that anything was possible.

When I began the diet, there was very little information available, so I started a Facebook group with a few friends who were trying fasting too – and when that group grew and grew (it now has over 20,000 members), I realised how powerful the 5:2 approach was. Group members were changing jobs, taking up exercise for the first time, even finding love; all thanks to their newly discovered confidence and sense of achievement.

I used that as the inspiration for a plan applying the same principles to all the things in life that influence our happiness and well-being. *5:2 Your Life* combines fun activities, great challenges and psychological research to create a very practical programme to help you transform your life – part-time!

How does *5:2 Your Life* work?

I designed the plan to take you through all the most important aspects of our lives – helping you to picture the life you want; improving your relationships; working fun fitness activities into your routine without joining a gym; and decluttering your home, your money and your mind.

The ideas and tasks are practical and proven, offering creative ways to help you feel happier and healthier. I've tried them all myself and I know the difference they make. I'm more confident, sleep better and am free from the winter blues that used to hit every year without fail.

There are no 'cookie cutter' solutions – this plan gives you the tools to work out exactly what *you* want the most – and the techniques to help you make changes you'll notice straight away.

Small changes, big dreams

All the activities in this book fit in around your life as it is now – you can work on your dreams during your daily commute, in your lunch break or once you've put the children to bed. Almost without noticing, you'll find that these little steps combine to produce a powerful ripple effect that will be felt all week long – and beyond.

And if you didn't get time to finish a challenge or activity – there's no guilt. You simply pick up where you left off the next day.

The 5:2 Eating plan – delicious meals to help you control your weight

Even the busiest person will be able to find enough time to try the enjoyable, energising activities – and *5:2 Your Life* also has a brand new six-week Eating Plan that complements the lifestyle challenges: you could lose a stone/6kg or more in the first six weeks. You can choose to do the Life Plan and the Eating Plan together, or separately – it's all about what *you* want the most.

What are you waiting for? It's time to *5:2 Your Life.*

1

5:2
BASICS

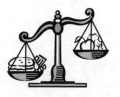

*What 5:2 is about,
why it works and
what you can expect*

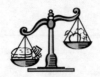

Small changes, big dreams

HOW 5:2 HELPS YOU TO TAKE CONTROL

Imagine the life you've always dreamed of.

OK. Let me qualify that a bit. Imagine the life that's like yours, but much, much better.

It's your life when the kids are getting on brilliantly and your partner gazes at you as though you're Brad Pitt/Angelina Jolie (if you're reading this, Brangelina, then, yes, 5:2 can even work for you). It's your life when you feel fit and positive: no health worries, no aches and pains, no looming bills you're struggling to pay. You love the work you do, and enjoy your leisure time and relationships. You sleep well, and wake up full of energy.

How does that life sound?

Maybe it's familiar – you have days like that already and you're hoping that 5:2-ing your life will give you more of them. Or maybe that sounds like an unattainable dream – or a very cheesy cereal advert. Perhaps you think that a life like that is only for the very lucky few.

Except luck is only a small part of the story. Most of the 'luckiest' people I know *seem* to glide through life, but in fact, they've put in the work and know where they're going. Just like a swan, effortlessly serene above the water, but paddling hard underneath.

You probably know there are things you could do right now that would help you make life better. But where would you start – and how on earth would you find the time? When there's work, and chores, and bills to be paid, and DIY jobs to be done, and people to be fed, the stuff that could make your life better never gets tackled. If you don't know where to begin, you never begin at all.

What if you could start small, by making changes just two days a week but feeling the positive effects all week long? What if each tiny change you made took you closer to the passions and the people that really matter to you?

That's *5:2 Your Life*, in a nutshell.

What does *5:2 Your Life* actually involve?

It's a six-week plan of enjoyable activities and ways to make your life better.

- **The 5:2 Your Life Plan** – a set of practical challenges and tasks to try out two days a week. Each week has a different theme – and includes an activity and a challenge using proven strategies to make you happier and more productive.
- **The Eating Plan** – based on the 5:2 Diet, this has satisfying meal plans for two fast days a week (don't worry – you won't be fasting completely!) plus advice on how to eat the rest of the time.

The 5:2 Life Plan themes

The themes for each of the six weeks have been chosen to enhance the areas of our lives that can promote happiness and well-being.

Week 1: Discover what matters to you and what you want to change – and begin to take action.

Week 2: Connect with the people you care about and the world you share.

Week 3: Simplify your life by getting rid of what's cluttering it up and tackling complications, especially finances.

Week 4: Move – make the mental and physical changes to increase your energy and happiness.

Week 5: Relax in the new space you've created and enjoy your free time.

Week 6: Do! – work out what you're best at and how to do more of it!

The plan is designed so that each week builds on the previous one – but you can choose to repeat a week, or do them in a different order. It's all about you!

Alternatively, if you have a real hatred of being told what to do, there's the DIY option:

DIY *5:2 Your Life*

You may want to choose this if you already have a really clear idea of the things you want to change – like giving up smoking, changing your job or decluttering your home. You'll design your own programme, using the tools in the book, to focus completely on that particular objective.

There's a separate chapter, DIY 5:2 Your Life (see page 255), to help you do that, selecting the best activities to work through on *your* 5:2 days.

Why part-time change works so well

Whether you follow the six-week programme, or design your own, the two-day approach is effective because:

1 You're **focusing your energies on small changes** and mini-goals that motivate you and keep you on track.
2 Change can be daunting – but committing to **making changes on just two days of the week is achievable.**
3 On the other five days, you're **seeing the benefits** of your 5:2 efforts – and you're also much more aware of the things you want to change, even when you're not specifically 'working' on them. So, almost without noticing, you'll probably start applying those same strategies beyond the two days – without feeling weak-willed or guilty if life gets in the way sometimes.

Why I know from personal experience that 5:2 is so much more than a 'diet'

5:2 has changed my life. As well as changing my body, it has changed my attitude to many aspects of my health and well-being. Yet it all started from watching a one-hour documentary in the summer of 2012.

But at this point I want to focus on the present. Right now:

- I'm 28 pounds (almost 13kg) lighter.
- I'm a UK size 10 (I was a 16.)
- My Body Mass Index (BMI – there's more about this in Part 3) is a healthy 22.8, rather than an overweight 27.6 – which should reduce the risk of conditions like Type 2 diabetes and some cancers . . .

- Yet I still bake every week, and enjoy smelly cheeses, great cocktails and meals out.
- I meditate regularly.
- I sleep better.
- I run or go to the gym twice a week and am much, much more active in my everyday life.
- I'm much less prone to the blues (one of the most significant improvements for me as I have suffered from depression in the past – I'll talk more about this in Part 2).
- I'm confident enough to go on TV and speak to international audiences about 5:2.
- I've achieved a lifelong ambition and written a cookbook.
- I've met more than 20,000 other 5:2 dieters online and in person.

and last but not least:
- I feel like part of a fantastic community – even, maybe, part of a revolution!

Others in our 5:2 Facebook group – where members share their weight loss and lifestyle tips and their amazing photographs and stories – have seen the same transformations. The results are much more far-reaching than looking better in a swimming costume (though that's a bonus). Here are some of the things they've achieved:
- Giving up smoking – probably the best thing you can do for your health – and your bank balance.
- Taking up running, cycling, Zumba, walking or gym classes for the first time.
- Setting themselves big challenges, like entering triathlons or fund-raising races.

- Cutting down on alcohol, sugar or other parts of their diet that they didn't feel were good for their bodies.
- Gaining the confidence to apply for – and get – new jobs.
- Spending more time with family and friends.
- Encouraging friends, family members and colleagues to make health improvements themselves.
- Feeling confident enough to buy new clothes that flatter them, or to fit into clothes they thought they'd never wear again.
- Taking up new hobbies, and going back to old ones, with the extra time and energy 5:2 has given them.

Many talk about 5:2 as a way of eating or a way of life, rather than a diet. They were motivated to make changes that went beyond what they ate – many using a free guide I put on my website at the end of 2012 about setting goals to improve your life. At the time, that was as far as I'd planned to go down the 'self help' route.

But when I began to hear the stories from the forums, I wondered how much more we could achieve by applying the 5:2 principles to some of the exciting techniques and research in the fields of positive psychology, mindfulness and life change.

Having shared this plan with guinea pigs from the groups, and seen them use the same simple principles to improve their lives, I know this 'diet' isn't just about making us slimmer.

It can make us *happier*, too.

2

THE

5:2

LIFE PLAN

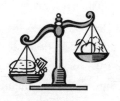

The practical, part-time way to work out what you want – and make it happen!

5:2 *Your Life* – the Life Plan

This part of the book contains all the activities and challenges for each of the six themed weeks to help you Discover, Connect, Simplify, Move, Relax and Do! See pages 257–271 if you want to go down the DIY route of designing your own plan.

Each week you choose two days to work through the activities. All the weeks follow the same basic pattern.

- **Introduction** to the week's theme.
- **Quiz** to make you think about the week's theme (optional, but fun to do!).
- On each of the two 5:2 days there is a:
  - **Key Activity** (often with a choice of options) – activities involve a mix of thinking, planning and taking action: they're divided into different steps, which take no more than 25 minutes in total.
  - **Challenge** – challenges involve doing something positive connected to that week's theme – they're usually energising and make an immediate difference.
  - **Bonus Activity** – for when you have the time to go a little deeper into the week's theme.
- **5:2 Inspirations** – indicated by the star symbol: research or studies to inspire you or make you think.
- **5:2 Myth-busting** – where we look at myths around each topic – for example, that you can't lose weight without taking exercise – and discover the truth.
- **Key points** – a summary of the week.

From Week 2 onwards, there's also a weekly 'checking in' page to help you monitor your progress.

Before you begin

What you need to *5:2 Your Life*

- Something to write in.
- Something to write with.
- Commitment to try out the activities.
- Time . . .

Ah, yes, *time*. That's the trickiest part.

The time factor

I'm always reading in the media about people who are 'cash rich, time poor'. And there are plenty of us who are also 'cash poor, time poor', of course. The good news is you don't need cash to 5:2 your life – but you will need to set aside time twice a week to try out the activities and challenges.

How much time depends on you, but as a guideline, each activity or challenge takes around 25-30 minutes. There are also optional extra ideas if you'd like to explore a topic more deeply, but on a 5:2 day, plan to set aside time for one activity and one challenge.

There are a handful of activities in the book where I *do* suggest trying to fit them in more often than twice a week. This might seem like I'm cheating! But the reason is always that research studies have shown those particular tools or tasks (including 'worry o'clock', meditation and expressive writing) work well when repeated several times in succession. It's very likely that they'll still produce great results when done two days a week – but to give you the best chance of success, I've always pointed out where there could be even greater benefits from more frequent repetition.

All the activities are designed to fit in around your everyday life and the existing demands on your time. **But you do have to want to try this. And I believe that where there's a will, there's a way...**

If two days is just too much, then you can do this one day a week – so the programme will take 12 weeks to finish. But it is important to try to fit in at least one activity or challenge each week – less than that, and it's likely you'll lose the momentum.

Hints for choosing days to *5:2 Your Life*

Choosing the right two '5:2' days will help improve your chances of success. If you're going to do the Eating Plan too, then doing the Life Plan on the same day can work – because you'll be spending less time preparing food or eating so may have time to spare! Plus it'll distract you from any tummy rumbles (especially on the first couple of fast days) – see Part 3 for guidance on how to plan your fast days.

So grab your diary/open up your computer calendar, and choose *two* 5:2 days in the coming week. If you can, plan ahead for the following six weeks, too. You can always change your days if you need to.

- Pick a day when you can build in some **time for yourself** (travelling, waiting to pick up the children, getting up a bit earlier).
- **Monday is a favourite day** to fast on the 5: 2 Diet - people love the idea of a fresh start and setting the tone for the week. The same can apply for 5:2 Your Life days.
- **Don't have two 5:2 days back to back** – it's best to have 'normal' days in between, to give yourself space to think about the tasks and have new ideas.
- If it suits you, **consider making the days the same each week**, so they become a routine.
- **That holiday feeling?** You might like to start the Life Plan on holiday – I always find I have a clearer perspective on the pluses and minuses of my life when I get away from the routine. And the exercises are fun to complete from the sunlounger – or in a tent as the rain pours down on the canvas.

Charting your 5:2 progress

The 5:2 Life Planner (see page 356) allows you to plot and plan your activities – and keep track of all you're doing and achieving. You can download a copy for printing out at the5-2dietbook.com.

Alongside the planner, you'll want a notebook and pen, or a tablet, smartphone or laptop with a note-taking function where you can work on the activities and challenges.

- A small notebook you can fit in your bag means you can take it everywhere in case inspiration strikes (I have a habit of getting a great idea staring out of a train window but then forgetting it by the time I'm back home!).

- If you're a visual person, it can enhance your creativity to use different coloured pens or pencils. (I love gel pens from Muji. Writing in purple changes my mood completely.)
- If you prefer using your phone or tablet, use an app like Evernote.com or a simple text app to jot down ideas and notes on the move – and transfer to a computer or print out later.

Finally, find a safe place to keep your notes, away from any nosy family members. You'll be more honest if you know no one else will read them!

Tell the world – or keep 5:2 a secret?

While we're on the subject of nosy people, who should you tell about 5:2?

One of the best ways to make this work is to find a 5:2 buddy – a supportive friend who'll do the activities at the same time and help you brainstorm!

Even if they don't want to 5:2 their own lives right now, it's great for you to have someone to talk to and brainstorm with. But choose a friend or family member who is likely to understand why you want to change the way you live your life or the way you eat. Occasionally, people can be unsupportive or be threatened by change, so pick a person who you think will understand what you're trying to achieve.

A great alternative is to join an online community. Many people swear by Facebook groups – and I've seen thousands of people succeed with encouragement from our 5:2 Diet group there. Nothing you post there appears on your timeline, but you do need to be happy to share your experiences with others on the same journey. I've set one up for this book on Facebook at facebook.com/groups/52yourlife – it's very much a self-help community where we can share ideas and experiences of the plan.

Highs and lows...

All the activities are designed to be both fun *and* challenging – but whenever we take a look at our lives, painful memories or difficult decisions can surface.

A little sadness can actually be productive – we can learn from our mistakes and regrets – but if you find that the exercises affect your mood for days at a time, then this may not be the right time for you to do the Life Plan. I've suffered from depression and I know there's a big difference between feeling regretful about the past, and the deeper feelings of despair and worthlessness that depression can bring.

Don't hesitate to ask your GP for help if you are feeling consistently low. There are also resources later to help you understand if you'd benefit from specialist help. But for most of us, the mood-boosting activities each week can make a big difference to how we feel!

What are you waiting for?

Week 1

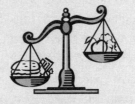

It is never too late to be what you might have been.

George Eliot

DISCOVER

THIS WEEK'S AIM:
**to discover what really matters to you –
and begin to make changes**

Introduction

We're kicking off the Life Plan with two 5:2 days devoted to discovering what matters most to you. It's an inspiring, fun introduction to this approach to life.

You might think that you already know what matters – but the activities this week can be revealing *and* surprising. On Day 1, you'll pinpoint the things that matter to you, and on Day 2, you'll map out your route, as all discoverers do, to improve your chances of uncovering the treasure at the end of your journey…

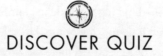

DISCOVER QUIZ

Each week, we start with an optional quiz, as a light-hearted way to get you thinking about this week's themes. If you hate quizzes, feel free to skip these – it's your (5:2) life, after all!

This week: **what your life is like right now.**

1   How does your adult life compare to the life you hoped for
    when you were a child?
    A   It's about what I expected – there are good days
        and bad days but generally I'm achieving the things I
        wanted to.
    B   It's worse: I'm pretty disappointed with the decisions
        I've made or some of the things that have gone wrong.
        I want to make things better.
    C   It's incredibly different – and much better. I feel lucky,
        but I've also worked hard, and keep working at it.
    D   I didn't know what life I'd end up living. I'm not
        much of a planner – I tend to leave things to fate, or
        circumstance.

2   Do you have a to-do list?
    A   Yes, and I sometimes even do the things on it!
    B   Yes, but it mainly reminds me of what I'm failing to
        achieve.
    C   Of course! In fact, I have more than one – and a five-
        year plan to keep me on track!
    D   No. I prefer to be spontaneous and tackle things when
        they arise.

3   You've got something big to tackle in your life – changing jobs,
    planning a wedding, moving house. How do you tackle it?
    A   I'm fairly organised but there's always something I
        forget.
    B   Panic – I usually get it all done but often I'm too tired to
        feel a sense of achievement by the time it's over.
    C   I plan it like a military operation, though sometimes that
        means I miss some of the fun along the way.

D   I tend to leave it to other people – organising stuff is not my strong point. It's probably why some things never change…

If you found yourself drawn to…

Mostly As: you're like most of us – too much to do, too little time! This week's Discover activities and challenges will help you build on your good habits and focus on the things that really make a difference to your quality of life.

Mostly Bs: if you're feeling stuck, or tired, then you're in the right place to make changes. 5:2 won't overwhelm you, but you can begin to make changes without adding to your burden.

Mostly Cs: you're super-organised – but if you're always focused on the end result, you can miss the thrill of the ride itself. Discover will help you survey the landscape and encourage you to try new things.

Mostly Ds: you hate planning – but if you approach it in the right way, it doesn't have to cramp your style. Read on to find out how you can look ahead without losing your spontaneity.

DISCOVER DAY 1

Great expectations, great big to-do lists

When I was a kid, I couldn't wait to be a grown-up, and do grown-up stuff. Travel the world, fall in love, make my mark.

The trouble is, grown-up stuff isn't all it's cracked up to be. In fact, at times, life seems to be one long – and dull – to-do list. We've often lost sight of the dreams and hopes we had.

My life isn't even that complicated, compared to friends with kids and other responsibilities. Yet I feel bogged down. There are days when I manage to get on top of all the stuff that comes with being a grown-up in the 21st century. But then there'll be an urgent deadline, or damp-proofing work, or something will break in the house or the car, and that tidal wave of stuff will start building. Before I know it, I'll be drowning again.

In theory, life should be simpler these days, because we can pay our bills online and Google anything tricky. Yet our expectations get higher, too. In my twenties, I'd happily book a £99 last-minute holiday to Greece, not even knowing which island we'd end up on, never mind whether the accommodation had a roof. Now I spend almost as long on TripAdvisor as I do on the holiday itself, fretting about reviews that complain about thin walls or dangerous sunloungers.

When that happens, I have to make a deliberate decision to stop and remember what really matters: finding somewhere I can relax, read, enjoy the sun and spend time with my partner or friends.

That's what the Discover week is about – a brief 'holiday' from the boring stuff, to spend quality time concentrating on what *really* matters. No sunlounger or factor 50 required! I'm not saying you abandon chores or stop paying your bills, but for the next half hour or so, *give yourself permission to look at the bigger picture*. Later we'll break it down into smaller tasks, but right now, this is about THINKING BIG.

5:2 INSPIRATIONS

INSIGHTS FROM THE END OF LIFE

Australian nurse Bronnie Ware has spent years working with those who are close to death. Her compilation of 'deathbed regrets' became a sensation on the internet – do read her full article at inspirationandchai.com/Regrets-of-the-Dying.html – I really recommend it.

The five most common regrets were:

1. I wish I'd had the courage to live a life true to myself, not the life others expected of me.

2. I wish I hadn't worked so hard.

3. I wish I'd had the courage to express my feelings.

4. I wish I had stayed in touch with my friends.

5. I wish that I had let myself be happier.

Bonnie's article ends by saying: *Life is a choice. It is YOUR life. Choose consciously, choose wisely, choose honestly. Choose happiness.*

Keep that in mind as you start your first activity. Ready to go? This activity is in two parts and will help you to start your journey of discovery . . .

Key Activity, Discover Day 1
Step 1
Find your 5:2 focus

You'll need:
- something to write on.
- a phone with a stopwatch, or a kitchen timer, to keep you focused.

Step 1:
This first part of this activity has four options.
   Option A: The bucket list.
   Option B: When I grow up.
   Option C: Picture your dreams.
   Option D: The big birthday party.

Simply choose the exercise that appeals to you most right now (you can always try the others at a later date)! These activities encourage you to 'brainstorm' – which basically means generating lots of ideas, including the craziest ones you can think of. It's important when you do this that you don't judge or dismiss any ideas, because the wackiest thoughts can lead to surprising and exciting plans and goals.

Whichever option you choose, it'll take around 15 minutes to complete before we move onto the second step.

Option A The bucket list

If you've never come across the phrase before, a bucket list is a list of things you'd like do before you die (or... kick the bucket!). Hopefully that's not happening any time soon, but in view of the deathbed regrets above, it can be revealing to start a list of the things you've longed to do.

- Find a quiet place to sit, take five slow, deep breaths and focus on feeling comfortable and relaxed.
- Set your phone alarm or kitchen timer for 15 minutes – and start writing your bucket list!
- If you need some ideas, think about:
  - Places – countries, cities, buildings or monuments to see, wildlife to witness, landscapes or geography to explore.
  - People – who do you want to meet or spend time with?
  - Activities – do you want to swim with sharks, sing in a band, skydive, make a film, take part in a triathlon? On a grander scale, do you want to fall in love, build a home, become a parent?
  - Events: whether it's Glastonbury, the Rio Carnival or the Verona Opera Festival, what are the must-see events for you?

- Legacies: what difference would you like to make, or what do you want to be remembered for? Charity work, the things you've created or made, the meals you've cooked?
- With any kind of brainstorming, it's often the ideas nearer the end of the session that are most surprising and interesting. So keep going even if you aren't finding it easy.
- If you want more ideas, visit bucketlist.net to discover what other people want to do!
- Got your list? Skip the other options and go to the second step of the exercise on page 32.

Option B When I grow up…

This activity is designed to help you tune into the passions and interests of the younger you, when you thought *anything* was possible.

- Find a quiet place to sit, take five slow, deep breaths and focus on feeling comfortable and relaxed.
- Set your phone or alarm for 15 minutes. Now close your eyes, and imagine yourself as a child, perhaps in a place where you used to daydream. The age you think back to doesn't matter, though try to focus on times before teenage self-consciousness kicked in.
- Think about the person you were then – your dreams, ideas, passions, hobbies, even crushes.
- Now begin to think about the things you hoped for back then.
  - **Routine:** What did you think your days as an adult would be like?
  - **Job:** Did you plan to be an astronaut, an artist, a vet?

- **Home Life:** Did you want to be a parent yourself? Where did you imagine yourself living? By the sea, in a city, abroad? And what kind of home did you picture?
- **Freedoms?** Did you dream of being able to choose to see movies without asking permission, or curling up with a book, or playing football for a pub team like your father?
- Scribble down any words or phrases that crop up. If you like, draw a picture. Or try writing with your non-dominant hand (i.e. the left, if you're right-handed), as it can take you back to that 'child like' feeling.
- All done? Got your list? Skip the other options and go to the second step of the exercise on page 32.

Option C Picture your dreams

A good option for creative types, anyone who thinks visually – or loves getting their hands dirty. You'll need pens, crayons or pencils or a pile of lifestyle/women's magazines and glue and scissors, and a big piece of paper. Just like being back at primary school…

- Take a large sheet of paper, and sit down at your biggest table. Spread out the pens, crayons or pencils or your selection of magazines.
- Set your phone or alarm for 15 minutes and draw your dreams – or make a collage by tearing and cutting stuff out of magazines (the collage option may take a little longer…).
- **If you're drawing,** remember the quality of your drawings is *totally* unimportant – what you want is to enjoy being free to make marks on the page, and do it fast! Think about the:
  - place where you'd like to live and kind of home you'd love.

- people (and animals) you'd like around you.
- job you'd like to be doin.g
- things you'd like to be doing in your leisure time.
- way you'd like to dress, look and feel.
- **If you're doing a collage,** flick through the magazines and tear out pictures and pages that appeal to you. But *don't overthink it* – it's more about mood and emotional response than consumer items.
  - Look at colours and landscapes and interesting people, rather than consumer items you want to buy or own.
  - Once you have a pile of images, lay them out on the page in different ways until you find an arrangement that appeals to you. Again, go on instinct rather than thinking it through too much.
  - Try out combinations that inspire you, or make you smile.
- Whether you're doing a drawing or a collage, do cover more than one page if you have time and the ideas are flowing… And remember you can keep adding to your drawing or collage – keep an eye out for images that appeal to you as you read during the six weeks of the plan!
- Finished your masterpiece? Skip the other options and go to the second step of the exercise on page 32.

Option D The big birthday speech

This exercise involves asking yourself lots of searching questions…
- Find a quiet place to sit, take five slow, deep breaths and focus on feeling comfortable and relaxed.

- Now think ahead to your next *big* birthday. You know the ones – they tend to end in 5 or 0. If you're within two years of a big birthday, skip ahead to the one *after* that (if you're 29, then choose 35; if you're 54, then go for 60!).
- Imagine it's the night of your birthday and you're having a great party. Jot down notes in answer to these questions:
  - Where is the party – which location, what venue? Who is coming?
  - Someone is giving a speech in your honour. Who is it – someone currently in your life, or a new person (partner, employer)?
  - What are they saying about you, your qualities, what you've achieved so far in your life?
  - What's happened between now – as you're writing – and this birthday to make this a reality? Think of the achievements that your speaker is describing.
  - How do you look and feel? Yes, you're older – but are you wiser, fitter and happier?
  - How do you respond to the speech? Think of who you'll thank for their part in your life.
- If you've finished imagining the party itself, then imagine the home you're going back to, and how you'll spend the day after your birthday: at work, enjoying a busy retirement, with your family?
- Enjoyed that? Now go to Step 2.

Key Activity, Discover Day 1 Step 2

The first part of the activity was about dreaming. I hope that whichever option you chose, it made you think! If you found it a little strange, that's normal – we rarely give ourselves permission to dream but it's highly recommended.

Now for part 2, we're going to be a little more analytical: this step is the same, whichever option you chose in part 1.

- Read through – or look at – your notes or pictures or collage. They might make you smile, or feel a bit sad, or both. That's normal!
- Take a new pen or highlighter and mark words or phrases that jump out at you:
  - Dreams or ambitions you'd forgotten.
  - Places or things you'd love to go to or do.
- If your ideas were based on images, then create a list of words to go with them. Focus on the emotions and common themes.
- Pick two or three of the keywords, priorities or ideas that seem important or are recurring:
  - Brainstorm them – think about whether there are elements you could incorporate into your life, or work towards.
  - A childhood dream of becoming an astronaut might be a tall order, but looking for a job with more travel or buying a telescope and trying out astronomy with your children is more than possible.
- For now, write down three *major* ideas or phrases that seem

particularly exciting or appealing. Keep them in a place where you'll see them – in your purse/wallet or notebook, or typed as a screensaver on your phone.

- Even if nothing very definite jumps out at you as something you can act on right now, you'll probably keep having ideas over the next few days. Remember to write them down!

As an example, when I did the Bucket List option, I wrote down about 30 different things – but the list of important themes that emerged was shorter: I ended up with ideas around travelling to countries I've never visited; cooking more (perhaps with ideas from my travels); being more ambitious with my own writing; and making a difference somehow.

So, I picked images of Australia to add to my laptop screensaver – and wrote 'make a difference' at the top of my daily to-do list, so I'd always be reminded about that before tackling the everyday tasks.

Oh, and my final one was very simple but the plans are still in hand: get a puppy!

Now's a good time to take a break. You've earned it! Grab a cuppa, take a stroll to the office water cooler or head off to take the dog or yourself round the block.

Key Activity
feedback – dreams and reality

Many people find it uplifting to imagine a better life, or to reconnect with past dreams. But it can be unsettling or uncomfortable at first if you're not used to looking at your life in this way.

Yet it's what many of the world's most successful and happiest people do. When people talk about 'goal-setting', it sounds very corporate, yet I think of 'goal' as just another word for a step towards achieving your dream. And there's plenty of evidence that goal-setting can help you get to where you want to be!

5:2 and the power of a shopping list

Sometimes getting what you really want starts with writing it down.

It's a bit like going out to do the grocery shopping. If you go to the supermarket without a list, you might get lucky and end up coming back with what you need, but it's much more likely you'll be distracted by special offers and end up with a bagful of stuff you didn't really want.

Whereas taking a couple of minutes to write a list before you leave means you'll probably spend less, save time and end up with what you need.

You can see life as a giant supermarket. Millions of choices and distractions that keep you from working out what you really want. Doesn't it make sense to stop and work out what your priorities are? Then, by focusing on those rather than the distractions that ambush you, you'll stand a much better chance of ending up with the life you really want.

GOOOOAL!

Setting goals doesn't mean everything will work perfectly – as John Lennon said, 'Life is what happens to you while you're busy making other plans.' But it certainly makes it easier to make choices – including the tiny ones you face every day – that support the aims and dreams you've decided to prioritise.

5:2 MYTH-BUSTING

THE FAMOUS GOAL-SETTING STUDY THAT NEVER HAPPENED

If you've read self-help books in the past, you might have come across a 1953 study that talks about a group of graduates from the prestigious Harvard University who wrote down their goals and were 'proven' in follow-up studies to have been way more successful (97% more, according to one report) than their peers. Inspiring, eh?

The only problem? The research doesn't exist.

I was pretty shocked by this when I couldn't find a trace of the study – it is quoted in many books and all over the web. However, there is a much smaller study by Dr Gail Matthews at Dominican University in California (see Resources, page 352 for a link) which shows that people who wrote down their goals, shared them with someone else and then sent weekly updates to that person were 33% more successful than those who just wrote goals down.

The Dominican study is not as compelling a study as the elusive Harvard one. But I do believe that goal-setting – and evidently, goal-sharing – can make a difference. It's worked for me, and for many others I know.

Challenge, Discover Day 1
what's in my way?

5:2 principles: small changes, big dreams

In the key activity, you worked out what you want to focus on over the next six weeks. You now know what you want more of in your life.

So why aren't you living that life already? Our next step is to work that out. We're going to see if we can identify what's standing in your way – so you can make plans to push through the barriers and take action. Yes, it can be challenging – but then that's the point of a challenge!

There are three options this time:

Option A: Draw the obstacles.

Option B: SWOT analysis.

Option C: Worry o'clock.

Take a quick look through and see which appeals most.

Option A Draw the obstacles

Even if you don't feel like an artistic person, this challenge can be very liberating indeed. (I'll share how I got on with this one later – it was pretty dramatic!)

- Get a large piece of paper and something to draw with – a big bold colour crayon or pen works well, or even charcoal.
- If you like, find some funky, feisty music and play it loud.

Set a timer for 15 minutes.

- Now fill the page with images of the things that stand in the way of you getting what you want. Don't worry about your drawing ability, or even if the images mean anything to you, just draw as fast and as freely as possible. Think about shapes, objects, people and fears, and try to represent them visually. Be big and bold!
- Once you've filled the page, take 10 minutes to review your drawing. How do you feel about it? You might find some surprising images on there.
- Getting the obstacles down like this can be emotional and powerful – but getting your fears on paper gets them out in the open. After you've finished, it's up to you whether to get rid of the page (you could rip it up or burn it – in the garden, obviously, if naked flames are involved), as a symbolic way of getting rid of the barriers… or keep it to see if it makes things clearer.

Option B SWOT analysis

This approach appeals to people who like a problem-solving and analytical approach. It comes from the business world and not everyone finds the management-speak headings very appealing, but if you're a methodical person, they can prompt useful questions and thoughts!

- Look at the keywords or ambitions that came out of the key activity. Choose one thing you'd love to do or achieve.
- Take a sheet of A4 and draw two lines to divide it into four squares, then put the headings in to match the squares shown over the page.

Strengths	Weaknesses
Opportunities	Threats

- Spend **5 minutes (set a timer) brainstorming each of the squares** in turn, in relation to your aim or ambition. *For example, if you'd love to run a half-marathon, your sheet might look like this…*

Strengths	Weaknesses
Loved running at school.	Youngest is only nine months – am I strong enough?
Very determined.	Prone to knee injury.
Really want to do it at the moment.	Tend to start things but then lose interest.

Opportunities	Threats
Half marathon coming up in our town next spring.	Money: don't have much money for clothes and gear.
Great woods to run in near where I live.	Knowledge: no idea how to train for a longer run.
Have a friend who did the half-marathon last time.	Time: I don't have much!

- Now, spend 5 minutes each finding practical solutions to only the weaknesses and the threats you've identified from the grid.

Weaknesses

Youngest is only nine months – am I strong enough?

Have a check-up with nurse at surgery; Google support and info online about new mothers who run; join an online forum?

Prone to knee injury

Go to local running shop to ask about supports before I start running instead of waiting for pain to start; think about speedwalking the race if need be.

Tend to start things but then lose interest

Use this as an experiment in keeping my interest sustained; vary my runs; make a great playlist; run with friends or in a group (ask at running shop)?

Threats

Money: don't have much money for clothes and gear

Prioritise – it doesn't matter what I run in for training, the trainers are the priority. I find the best value shop and put money aside each week for any extra I need for race itself.

Knowledge: no idea how to train for a longer run

Ask friend who has done it to take me through it; download an app to my phone and run with that.

Time: I don't have much!

Can I build the running into other activities – run the long way to pick up the kids from school, run around the area where Mum lives while she babysits, ask Andrew to look after them all for an extra hour on Sunday while I train?

Option C Worry o'clock

Anxiety has always served a purpose for humans – it's kept us safe from danger by making us aware of hazards, from predators to thunderstorms. But if our worries begin to take over, and our fears become irrational and out of proportion, they become counter-productive.

The 'worry o'clock' approach was pioneered in the 1980s and is based on a psychological idea known as 'stimulus control'. The aim is to change how you respond to a worry or 'stimulus.' A recent study from the Netherlands shows it can be effective for people who are anxious (see Resources from page 352 for a link to the research). This is a technique you can use if you find that anxiety and worries preoccupy you day after day.

The idea is to schedule worrying time into your day. Outside that time, you simply take a note of the worry then postpone it. When worry time comes, you'll be focussed on finding solutions and ready for action.

This is one of those occasions that I suggest bending the 5:2 rules: the research that found it effective was based on scheduling worry time every night. So, if you have time to do it for several evenings in a row, you may see faster results.

- **Start a worry list:** whenever you recognise that you're beginning to worry, stop. Take out your list, write down the worry – a few words, no more – and tell yourself you are going to set a schedule time to worry about it later, at a set time. Then simply return to what you were doing before the worry started.

- **Set worry o'clock:** choose a specific time on your 5:2 day for worrying (not just before you go to bed). Aim for 20 minutes solid!

- **At worry o'clock:** set a timer for 20 minutes. Take out your list and focus on the worries, but try your hardest to move beyond simply worrying, and towards problem-solving. (You could try the SWOT exercise on page 37, the financial and money-saving tools from pages 133 to 134, or the tips on creating better habits on page 170 to help find solutions.)

- **Keep your appointment on your 5:2 nights – preferably each night if you can** – for at least a week. The more often you do it, the more likely you are to get very bored with having to keep the appointment… which is part of the point: we want to make worry boring, but also focus the mind on finding solutions rather than going in anxious circles.

You might find that having an appointment once a week, or a short 5-minute slot daily, will help you in the medium term, but many people find it does simply reduce worries overall and focus the mind on finding solutions.

Postponing worries means you can get on with your everyday life, but know you'll have time to tackle the important issues when you're in the right frame of mind. Once you have your list, you can be clearer about what really needs to be dealt with – like tackling debt or dealing with health issues – and pointless worries, like fretting about the odd grey hair …

Challenge: feedback

How did you find the challenge you chose? I've tried them all and they're useful in different ways. But I thought I'd share my own experience of the drawing exercise…

The power of drawing obstacles: my experience

I am really bad at drawing. Art was the only exam I failed at school and I've had a bit of a complex about it ever since…

In 2012 I decided to do an adult education class based on a book called *The Artist's Way* by Julia Cameron, which is all about being more creative, in all aspects of your life. It's a book and an approach I do recommend – there are more details later in this book (see page 80).

At the time, I was feeling quite unsure about my own writing.

I'd achieved my dream of writing a novel. In fact, I'd written ten – a couple had been bestsellers and the others had been nominated for awards. Yet I was feeling stuck. Afraid about whether I could manage it again. Burned out, really.

The class was fun, the people supportive, and the activities were a mix of the inspiring and the scary. That afternoon, our tutor told us to draw our fears and what was holding us back.

My fear at that exact moment was drawing *anything*. But I picked up some charcoal and a large sheet of paper and began to draw.

Within a few short minutes I'd filled the page – there were closed doors, graveyards and tombstones, which seemed to represent the end of my creativity or my career. There were laughing faces and words like FAILURE and POVERTY and RUBBISH.

It was surprising *and* upsetting. The tutor invited us to tear up our pictures and throw them away, but I wasn't ready to, even though the images were negative.

That night, I looked at the images again. It was strange but I suddenly felt less scared. The pictures showed what I was afraid of – failure, mockery, humiliation – yet picturing them helped put them in their place. I realised that writing involved risk – but that I loved it too much to give it up. Plus I began to make a back-up plan to pay the bills if my income took a hit.

I don't think it's coincidence that within a week of doing the drawing, I had the idea to write the book I couldn't find when I started doing 5:2 dieting… the book that has changed so much in my life for the better and introduced me to some amazing people.

I can't promise that the activities will have as dramatic or immediate an effect on you. But I do know that what you

43

started today will open your mind to new ways of thinking, seeing the world and living.

'Whether you think you can or think you can't – you're right'

Car giant Henry Ford is famous for this quote, which emphasises how our thoughts can strongly affect the results we achieve. But as today's challenge shows, I don't think it's realistic to ignore the negatives or obstacles standing between us and our dreams.

Instead, becoming aware of the issues we're facing means we're often in a far better position to find a solution that will actually work.

We're almost done with today – I hope the activities have given you lots of food for thought. Our final activity is optional – but it's a great reward for your hard work as it's all pleasure, and no pain!

Bonus Activity, Discover Day 1: the pleasure list

When was the last time you did something purely for yourself that made you feel great?

This activity is all about rewarding yourself! I've adapted it from a technique used in Cognitive Behavioural Therapy, which helps people change their thinking and raise their mood. The particular technique used is known as Activity Scheduling, where people are encouraged to schedule time to do things they enjoy.

It's that simple!

Step 1

- Start a pleasure list – right now, write down ten things you could do for yourself that would make you feel good.
- You could create two lists – one for free treats or pleasurable activities; one that may involve spending some money. Here are some examples:
  - Free pleasure: give yourself 20 minutes to read a book or magazine (either in the bath or in your favourite chair with a mug of hot chocolate); watch your favourite sports on TV; do your own hand massage and manicure; take a walk in the park; make up a new 'happy' playlist from your old tracks; watch a comedy you love online.
  - Paid-for treats : have a massage or treatment (local colleges with beauty departments often offer cut-price treatments); book afternoon tea with a friend or on your own; go for a night out with mates to the pub.
- Keep your pleasure list handy. Add to it as new ideas come to you during the week. You can *never* have too many treats.

Step 2

- Choose one of those pleasurable activities to do today – or, if you've run out of time, squeeze in a treat before your next 5:2 day. Choose when you'll do it and write it on your Life Planner or in your diary/calendar right now!
- When you've had your treat, jot down how it made you feel – and whether it's one you'd like to do again soon, or if

45

it gave you some new ideas for future pleasurable activities, which you can add to the list.

Why treats matter

There is something a bit 'women's magazine' about the treat task. I love women's magazines but sometimes the suggestions – the hot bath, the manicure – seem glib or patronising...

But there's more to treating yourself than the activity you choose. I believe very strongly that we need to treat ourselves as we treat others – with kindness and understanding.

The idea of treating yourself might seem uncomfortable at first – as though it'll make you self-indulgent or weak somehow. The truth is, many of us lack confidence or don't feel great about ourselves. Giving ourselves mini-rewards or nice things is one way to make us feel more deserving... which could even make us luckier in life...

5:2 INSPIRATIONS

I SHOULD BE SO LUCKY...

Psychologist Richard Wiseman has spent much of his career studying luck – and believes people create it for themselves (see more on his site at richardwiseman. wordpress.com). He also thinks you can become luckier, partly by simply believing you are more likely to get lucky... People who believe they're fortunate, will make it happen by:

- expecting good things to happen to them and tending to keep going till they get the positive result they expected all along;
- noticing chances and opportunities by being open to new experiences and being in contact with people who can make things happen;
- listening to their instincts – we all have hunches but luckier people are more aware of them and more likely to act on them reacting to bad fortune by moving on quickly and taking control.

DISCOVER DAY 2

Checking in

Welcome back! Have the exercises you did on Day 1 given you new ideas and made you see your life differently? That's normal, and can be a bit unsettling – but writing down the feelings and experiences does help.

If you're doing the plan at the same time as a friend, or are a member of our Facebook group, then do share your discoveries as you make them!

Getting your priorities right – what matters most?

Today we're going to focus on how to turn the insights you discovered on Day 1 into practical steps to make you happier: in other words, how to **get your priorities right!**

The activities on Day 1 often reveal a conflict between the big priorities in your life – relationships, career, health – and the more trivial stuff that clutters up our to-do lists.

It's the battle of the big stuff vs the small stuff.

Not sweating the small stuff (and the cost of a breakdown)

You might have heard of the book, *Don't Sweat the Small Stuff* – it was a big hit a few years back. The idea is that we waste too much time focusing on the small stuff like paperwork and chores and petty issues, and it's one I agree with... up to a point. Sorting out insurance might seem 'small' but it pretty soon turns big if you have a bump in the car or your house burns down.

But we can end up letting the small stuff dominate. An example: I am addicted to the UK website moneysavingexpert. com – I have a lifelong fear of debt and so I'm always scouring the site for the cheapest deal. The downside – it can take *hours* to make any little decision.

This year, when it came to renewing my breakdown insurance (pretty essential as my Ford Ka is now 13 years old), I decided to weigh up the saving I might make against the amount of time it would take me to change companies, which I usually do: it would involve researching the alternative breakdown cover, cancelling the direct debit, setting up a new one, making sure I'm not paying for two services by accident... I have been really busy with bigger stuff – like writing this book – and I suddenly wondered if it was worth the hassle.

And I decided to let it auto-renew...

We'd had good service from the company this year, nice helpful patrols who've got us going after two breakdowns. I could have saved £25 by switching – and there are times when I've needed to save that last £25 more than save time – but this year I decided to prioritise.

It might not sound like a big decision, but for me, with my anxieties around money, doing that felt daring... and quite liberating.

Now it's your turn. There's only one option for this next activity, because it will work for everyone!

Key Activity, Discover Day 2
take 10!

Step 1 – 10 minutes

- Take your notebook or smartphone/tablet/laptop. Write 'Big Stuff' at the top of one page and 'Small Stuff' at the top of the second.
- Set your alarm for 5 minutes and write down all the large-scale tasks you're facing at the moment, both exciting and stressful. They might include moving house, changing career, planning for retirement: complex or long-term items, including the kind of things you thought about on Day 1.
- Now take another 5 minutes to scribble down the small stuff: think about clutter that's built up around the home, the mouldy shower curtain, the final changes of address you haven't got round to two years after moving, switching your broadband or mobile contract, sewing on buttons that have fallen off the kids' coats.

Step 2 – 10 minutes

- Look at the 'small stuff' list. And pick something to tackle, right now. Something you can do in 10 minutes.
- Go and do it! Set your alarm… see you in 10!

Step 3 – 10 minutes

- Done it? Great! Don't lose the momentum. In your notebook, start a 'take 10' list – jot down ten more things that will take you 10 minutes or less to achieve. I think them as my whirlwind tasks.
- Resolve that you will tackle one 'take 10' item each 5:2 day (or every day if you're feeling keen). Each time you complete one, record it on your planner, to keep track.
- If you're feeling overwhelmed during your day, or paralysed by the number of things you have to do, turn to the list and tackle something on it without delay. I promise it's a great way to feel less like a procrastinator and more like a doer!

Key Activity
feedback – how do you feel?

I feel pretty good myself. Here's what I did: I went all out to clear out my Stationery Drawer from Hell.

It's the drawer in my desk that I use most often, and the one that drives me crazy. It annoys and frustrates and irritates and guilt-trips me as it's a nest of rechargers, staples, envelopes, stamps, pens and grubbiness. Here's what I did:

- Set the clock for 10 minutes.
- Tipped the lot onto my desk.
- Cleared out all the grubbiness (pencil marks, rusty paperclips, hair?!) with an anti-bacterial wipe.
- Chucked all the random things in the bin – the ear buds from old personal stereos that don't fit, the pencil from IKEA that's too small to write with (though I felt a bit guilty).
- Attached the back-up external hard drive I found under the envelopes to my computer.
- Put the receipts I haven't had time to file in an envelope.
- Put everything back in sections (top tip from my boyfriend is to reuse well-washed plastic takeaway containers to organise your drawers – or buy new containers from the pound shop).
- Enjoyed the rosy glow from my new, super-streamlined Stationery Drawer from Heaven.

The key to this was *definitely* doing it fast. I could have spent longer but the whirlwind approach to getting things done at speed was really satisfying – and as this is the drawer I open most often, it's going to give me a buzz each time I do!

Putting the small stuff in its place: why whirlwinds work

Maybe you think it's weird that I've been banging on about tackling huge life change – and now I'm telling you to spend 10 minutes dealing with trivia. But the speed/beating the clock element is the point – it stops deliberation and agonising over things that really don't merit too much thought. And leaves your brain clear to tackle the important things.

THE POWER OF THE POMODORO – OR GETTING ORGANISED, ONE TOMATO AT A TIME

My whirlwind approach is my own take on another technique that I love to use when I need to get focused. It's called the Pomodoro Technique (PT for short).

If you speak any Italian (even pizza menu Italian) you'll realise *pomodoro* means tomato – and when I tell you this approach is named after those retro tomato-shaped kitchen timers, you'll realise this isn't your average management technique.

The idea, first developed in the 1980s by Francesco Cirillo, is based on the principle that human beings can only focus for a certain period of time before their attention wanders. I think it varies from person to person, but the PT assumes that for most of us, the maximum time is 25 minutes. The principle is:

- If we can only focus for around 25 minutes at a time, let's break down everything we need to do with our day into 25-minute sections – and award ourselves a short 5-minute loo/stretch break at the end of each chunk.
- At the end of every four Pomodoros (which is what Cirillo calls those chunks), you get a proper break.

You can read much more about the PT online on Cirillo's website, http://pomodorotechnique.com. The theories are more complex than I am outlining here, and there are numerous charts and other tools you can use to plan your work and leisure time and monitor your progress.

What works best for me is a little app on my desktop that replaces the tomato timer, and it buzzes helpfully at the end of each 25-minute chunk (I currently have 12 minutes and 41 seconds of my second chunk of the day left). It's called the Pomodairo and I really recommend it – download it from http://pomodairo.en.softonic.com.

But, as my Take 10/whirlwind approach proves, you don't have to work in units of 25 minutes. It could be 10 or, if you have supreme concentration, 45. For me, the power of this kind of time-focused working comes from two things:

- Working against the clock helps me to focus on what's achievable, rather than the hugeness of a task (and I naturally seem to speed up as the clock ticks down!).
- It forces me to focus on one thing – and if I can't even focus for 25 minutes, then I am in a very bad way. (Admission: sometimes around the 14-minute mark I have the urge to check my email. I always resist. Well, *almost* always.)

The technique doesn't appeal to everybody, but it's one of the techniques I've shared that people always mention with a broad grin – even fellow authors, who are some of the best procrastinators I know.

The Pomodoro Technique is just one way to break big tasks into more manageable chunks. It's something we often do with physical activities – hardly anyone would do a triathlon without a training programme to build up stamina. Yet we don't often do it for things like job-hunting or finances.

PS: if you like the technique, treat yourself to a fun kitchen timer. I spent a whole Pomodoro's worth of time looking online for a timer, ending up with one that looks like a man in a Chinese outfit. Super-cute. But it's not very good at keeping time… whoops!

Bonus (Optional) Activity
shrinking the big stuff

This is an optional activity, but it's in tune with Pomodoro principles. We're putting this one before today's challenge, while the idea of dividing up your time is still fresh in your mind.

Step 1
- Look at your 'big stuff' list, and the list of dreams/ambitions from Day 1. Choose a task that you believe will make you happier. Maybe it's starting your own business, because that's on your bucket list – or it could be a charity bike ride in Asia for a cause that means a lot to you. Choose something ambitious that excites you.
- Spend a minute or two imagining yourself achieving this aim in a year's time. Picture how you'll feel and what you'll be doing – crossing the finish line, handing over the fund-raising cheque, working on your own stall or updating your business website with news of an award you've just won.
- Now brainstorm on paper all the steps that you'd need to take to get there. So, for example:

* For the business, you'd need a business plan, time to devote to developing your product or service, funding for any start-up equipment, a marketing plan/website, space in your home or outside it to develop it, perhaps new arrangements at work or support from family so you can put the hours in.
* For the bike ride, you'd need to find the right event and dates, work on a training schedule, investigate travel and costs, perhaps find the money for a new bike and organise sponsorship.

Step 2

Right now, that might look a bit overwhelming. But every runner or entrepreneur has felt like that at the start of their journey – and learned to ignore it!

- Choose just **one of those steps or stages** – preferably the first one – and break what needs to be done down into 25-minute chunks. **For the bike ride,** finding the right event could take a couple of 25-minute sessions:
  * looking online for the right charity and an event taking place at the right time
  * registering
  * researching accommodation and travel costs
  * considering which friends or family might join you.
- Once you've tackled the first step, move onto the next, e.g. training. This will be the biggest part of your preparation, but you can break it down into:
  * finding a structured training plan online, in a magazine or from a friend
  * finding a cycling club
  * working out training routes

* looking at your diary for good times to train.
- In the **business example**, marketing is a huge task, but you can begin to break it down into:
  * researching online how any competitors market their products – and what you like/don't like
  * setting up an online survey asking friends where they hear about similar products
  * setting up a Twitter account for the business name
  * researching website designers – or finding a simple package you could use yourself.

Step 3

Commit to do at least two Pomodoros towards your goal in the coming week. If you have time, then start right now! It won't happen overnight – but spending just an hour or two a week on the bigger picture will take you closer to your dreams…

What if I hate tomatoes? (And tomato-sized goals)

The Pomodoro Technique isn't the answer for everyone, or to every problem. Even as a big fan of goal-setting, I know there are times when it feels better to jump straight into sorting out an issue, or to act on instinct, rather than analysing an issue in depth. Especially as life doesn't often go exactly to plan…

Dwight Eisenhower said that 'In preparing for battle, I have always found that plans are useless but planning is indispensable.' And this from the man who helped make D-Day happen. Embrace that – the world is uncertain, but if we've thought something through in advance, we're prepared for action.

And keeping your plans in mind has another, unexpected advantage...

5:2 INSPIRATIONS

THE PUPPY EFFECT

Your brain isn't always the most reliable judge of what's true and what's not – psychologists have been studying what are called 'cognitive biases' for many years and generally they're seen as unhelpful because they give you a false picture of the world. But sometimes you can make them work in your favour. I'm calling this example the 'Puppy Effect.'

Right now, we're thinking of getting a puppy – and now every time I go out, I seem to see them! They have appeared *from nowhere* with their wagging tails and eager faces.

Except they haven't appeared from nowhere at all... they were always there. It's just I am looking for them sub-consciously, and it *appears* that they're everywhere. It's one of those tricks your brain performs – giving you an illogical, but actually quite useful, view of the world. My Puppy Effect example is trivial – but it still helps me gain new information by observing different breeds and chatting to their owners. You might find the same if you're considering buying a car, or getting a new haircut – you suddenly notice the make or style everywhere.

All very interesting – but how can it help you change your life? The trick is to get your sub-conscious working for you, by creating reminders of your new goals or dreams. Those reminders will then help you spot opportunities you might not have seen otherwise.

That's what we're doing to do in our challenge – visualise your goals or put them into words:

Challenge, Discover Day 2
The Power of Dreams and Reminders

In this challenge, you're picking a priority or dream, making it more tangible – and then helping your conscious and sub-conscious mind to find ways to make it happen for real.

- Look at your lists of big stuff from today, and at the 'find your 5:2 focus' work you did on Day 1. Choose something that really excites you or matters to you.
- Now you want to find words, images or sounds to help you keep that ambition or dream in mind, and help it become more real and seem more possible. Ideally you'll see the reminder several times each day. Here are some ideas:

- **Images:** a picture of a place, an object or a person that reflects what you want to do or see or become. Or a photo of your completed collage or drawing if you made one to visualise your dreams.

- **Words:** it's good to condense your dream into a few vivid words, and in the present tense, too, as though you're already doing what you love. It feels strange, even boastful or fanciful at first but research suggests it can help make things happen – 'I run a thriving business baking delicious, fun celebration cakes' or 'I am going on an amazing world cruise to see all the sights I've dreamed of' or 'I spend lots of precious time every day doing things with and listening to my children.' An alternative is to find an inspiring quote from a person you admire.

  - **Where to see or read them:** both the images and words could go next to your bed, inside the kitchen cupboard or your wardrobe (taped to the back of the door), on the fridge or in your purse or wallet (in the clear pocket where your bus pass or Oyster card goes so you see them every time you open it). Or you could put them as the screensaver on your phone or laptop.

- **Sounds:** if you love music, then find an inspiring piece of music or a song to associate with your dream. Or if you want to travel to a place, or move home, find sounds from nature or locally produced music to create a soundtrack for your plans.

  - **Where to hear the sounds:** make it the first song on your playlists. Try finding it as a ringtone on your phone or as your alarm – and make the effort to play the song just before bed, too. Make the association clear by playing it while you are working towards fulfilling your ambition or living your dream.

- **Touch/scent:** objects can be a great reminder – especially natural objects like a tiny pebble or seashell to remind you of places where you might like to live or visit. If you like jewellery, then a charm or a pendant can be a physical reminder of something you want. Scent is a little more subtle and best combined with something more visible, but even a shower gel or perfume you used when you were younger, or on holiday, can be uplifting and has the advantage of being used often. Or choose fragrances or oils made in a place or way you find inspiring.

> **• Where to experience it:** if the object is small enough, carry it with you, or wear it as jewellery. People might ask about it, too, which gives you a chance to share your vision if you want to. Or, if it's larger, keep it on your coffee or bedside table: pick it up, feel the textures and the weight of it, and take a moment a couple of times a day to think about the idea associated with it. Use scents in your daily life, in an oil burner or diffuser.

A week of discovery – and the start of the adventure

That's the end of your first *5:2 Your Life* week – give yourself a pat on the back for making a start on something fantastic!

I hope you enjoyed it. Before you go, remember to:

- put next week's 5:2 days in your diary
- keep adding to your pleasure list if you started one on Day 1 (if not, try it now, it only takes a minute to begin a list of things you enjoy!)
- tackle a 'take 10' task every 5:2 day

- keep a note of any feelings or experiences or ideas that come to you during the week.

Discover Week: key points

Here's a summary of our key points from this week:

- Small actions can make a huge difference – and each step will take you closer to your dream.
- When you're really stuck, do something small but practical to get back the feelings of achievement.
- Planning won't necessarily make things go your way every time, but will help you feel prepared for whatever happens.
- Build reminders of your dreams and ambitions into your daily life.
- Treat yourself kindly!

Week 2

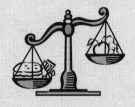

I've learned that people will forget what you said, people will forget what you did, but people will never forget how you made them feel.

Maya Angelou

Week 2: checking in

Each week, before we start our new theme, it's a great idea to take a couple of minutes to think about the impact of the previous week.

- Did the Discover activities and challenges trigger any particular thoughts or feelings after you'd finished? Memories, ideas, even occasionally sad feelings. Jotting them down in your notebook can help you feel better and understand your responses.

- Have you had more ideas about what you want to achieve and what's important to you? Your dreams *will* evolve and become clearer as you work through the Life Plan.

- Have you been trying out the Take 10/whirlwind approach (see page 54 for a reminder)? My tip is start close to you – which I literally did by sorting out my desk drawer. Next step: the Cluttered Admin Table of Doom…

CONNECT

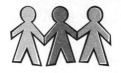

THIS WEEK'S AIM:
to connect more with the people who matter to you,
and with the world around you

Introduction

This week, we're going to work on how we relate to the rest of the world – in other words, how we connect to those we're close to, and to our community.

If that sounds woolly, I promise you it's anything but. Research on what makes us happy shows that feeling connected to other people and the place where we live is one of the most significant factors when it comes to feeling satisfied.

On Connect Day 1, we'll focus on practical steps to help us value and enjoy time spent with those we care about *and* spent alone. Becoming more aware of our emotions, our surroundings and our relationships with family and friends, can make a big difference to our everyday lives.

And on Connect Day 2, we'll look at how we fit into the wider world, and what we can do to feel we're making a difference.

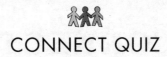

CONNECT QUIZ

As in week one, we start with a fun quiz to introduce you to this week's topics.

This week: **how you connect**

1   Picture the place where you live. How does it make you feel?

    A   Happy – I love my neighbours and can't imagine living anywhere else.

    B   Stressed – I'm worried about crime, noise and don't like being on the streets at night.

    C   Frustrated – I'd love to know more about my local area, and maybe help to make it better, but where do I find the time?

    D   Not that bothered – I don't tend to get involved as I move home often, and so do the neighbours.

2   When was the last time you had a proper conversation with a good friend – and felt you really listened to them and they really heard you?

    A   This week – I couldn't do without the chance to catch up and talk through what's going on with my life.

    B   This month – but I often feel either that we're both too wrapped up in our own issues to listen properly to the other person.

    C   It's on my to-do list, but we keep playing phone tag.

    D   I don't really have those conversations – I'm more likely to go out in a big group.

3   Do you support any charities or campaigns?
    A   Yes – I give regularly to a favourite cause, and try
        to volunteer when I can.
    B   I feel I should but the choice is so overwhelming
        and makes me feel guilty about the causes I'm then
        not supporting.
    C   I always sponsor colleagues and friends when they
        do an expedition, and would love to do something
        similar myself.
    D   I feel people need to look after themselves because
        we can't rely on charities or outside help.

If you found yourself drawn to…

Mostly As: you're connecting really well already – but this week will confirm why it's so important.

Mostly Bs: stress and anxiety may be getting in the way of feeling more connected, but all it takes is small steps to feel better. This week's activities can help you make the first move.

Mostly Cs: like most of us, you're pushed for time – but connecting more doesn't have to mean a huge commitment or lots of work. Read on for more ideas.

Mostly Ds: right now, 'connecting' isn't a priority. Of course, there's no law that says you have to be a pillar of the community. But you might be surprised by the difference it can make to your day-to-day life if you can feel closer to the people you're with, and the area where you live.

CONNECT DAY 1

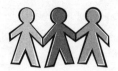

If you're happy and you know it, clap your hands?

Happiness is a funny thing. We spend our lives looking for it, and yet when we actually find it, we're often too busy enjoying life to realise it… it's only when things aren't going so well that we look back on the good times and understand what we had.

Well, this week, we're going to try to capture that elusive feeling – and nurture it.

You gotta accentuate the positive…

The positive psychology movement was founded by Martin Seligman and his team at the University of Pennsylvania in 1998. The idea behind the movement is to focus on practical things we can do to improve our mood and our sense of purpose in life.

One of the key messages is that enhancing our relationships and our sense of 'connection' with the world can add meaning to our lives. Yet it's so easy to take the important people for granted, or to neglect the things that make us happy.

Elements of happiness

What does happiness mean to you? Take a moment to jot down a few ideas.

Done it?

Let's see what the statisticians have to say…

5:2 INSPIRATIONS

WHO ARE THE HAPPIEST PEOPLE ALIVE?

You might think the keys to happiness are the qualities we see celebrated in magazines: youth, wealth, beauty.

But according to the World Happiness Database, the young, the rich and the beautiful don't have all the answers, thank goodness. It's more important to hang out with people you like, to live in an equal society and to be able to afford to go out for dinner now and then. Oh, and while it's nice to be pretty, how attractive you are is *less* important than how attractive you *think* you are!

According to a BBC report from July 2013 (see the Resources section from page 352 for the link), other factors that influence our happiness include:
- being in a long-term relationship
- being physically active at work and in your free time
- drinking alcohol in moderation (people who do this tend to be happier than those who don't drink at all)
- having close friendships (though the number of close friends isn't as important as the quality)
- being actively engaged in politics.

The politics one surprises me, but other studies have shown that being involved in your community helps increase satisfaction levels, so perhaps politics is simply another way to connect with like-minded people.

What about having children? Surprisingly, one study shows that they can lower your happiness levels – but that you *are* happier once they leave home…

And work? Obviously it's good to like your job, but the location of your work matters too. Commuting has a negative effect on your happiness – if you travel for over an hour each day, then you'll be less happy than those who don't commute. And, unfortunately, earning more because you're willing to travel won't make up for the loss of precious leisure time.

Location, location, location

Where you live in the world also affects your happiness – but again, you might be surprised. I assumed that the Mediterranean countries – famous for their great diet and climate – would top the list, but actually, four of the top five can be distinctly chilly:

1 Costa Rica
2 Denmark
3 Iceland
4 Switzerland
5 Norway

(Source: Countries ranked in order of 'satisfaction with life', according to the World Database of Happiness.)

From theory to real life...

For most of us, moving to Costa Rica isn't an option. So, how can we increase our happiness levels without emigrating?

The BBC decided to find out – by organising an experiment in 2005 that aimed to make an entire town happy. They chose the English town of Slough and their action plan was partly based on the Seligman positive psychology movement and research. Here is a list of their ideas:

Making Slough Happy – the suggestions

- Plant something and nurture it.
- Count your blessings – at least five – at the end of each day.
- Have an hour-long conversation with a loved one each week.
- Give yourself a treat every day and take the time to really enjoy it.
- Have a good laugh at least once a day.
- Get physical – exercise for half an hour three times a week.
- Smile at and/or say hello to a stranger at least once each day.
- Cut your TV viewing by half.
- Spread some kindness – do a good turn for someone every day.

Too simple? We'll be finding out be experimenting with similar ideas this week.

Guidance on re-connecting

Some of the exercises do involve taking a risk because you may be contacting people you haven't seen for a while, or trying to change how you relate to friends or family members. Of course, you can't always predict how others will respond – so our activity is about reaching out, while the challenge is about boosting your confidence from within.

Key Activity, Connect Day 1
reaching out

There are four options. Simply choose the option that appeals most.

Option A: Absent friends
Option B: The thank-you letter
Option C: Dinner for four (or three, five…)
Option D: Fairy godmother

Option A Absent friends

- Write a list of the people you've lost touch with or haven't seen much of lately/would like to see more of. I'm not talking about deep rifts, but people you like/would like to see more of/used to work with/live close to. Your mobile phone contacts list is a good start to help you remember.

- Pick five and send a text message, an email or even a postcard: we so rarely get anything fun in the post these days, so that could really raise someone's spirits when they discover it among the junk mail, the spam messages or the bills. Whether you're writing or texting, tell them you've been thinking of them. You could thank them for a good memory you shared.

- The trick is to contact several people at a time, so you don't feel too much is riding on one person's response.

Note: this may not be one for when you're feeling sad because not everyone may be in a position to reply – but if you want to rekindle some friendships and are feeling brave, the potential benefits make it worth taking the risk.

Option B The thank-you letter

- This activity is one that's often associated with positive psychology – and there's a reason why. Writing a letter to someone you care about to thank them for what they've brought to your life will create warm feelings for you *and* them.
- Choose someone you're grateful to – it could be a friend, family member, partner, mentor or even someone you've lost touch with or who has died.
- You can type this on a laptop, but I think pen and paper/a card is much nicer (though if you're anything like me, you'll be shocked at how bad your handwriting is these days).
- Allow yourself at least half an hour to write a thank-you letter to explain what you feel they've done for you, and why you appreciate them. Think about specific times and memories, but also the personal qualities you admire in that person. If you feel like it, add doodles or photos to the letter or the envelope.
- If you're still in touch, do consider sending the letter. But even if the person is no longer contactable, the chances are those memories have reminded you of happy times. Appreciate those feelings and the part that person has played in who you are now. You can keep the letter for when you want to remind yourself about the connection you had.

Option C Dinner for four (or three, five...)

- Commit to eat at the table with your family or partner twice this week (if you don't have a table big enough, then arrange a picnic on the floor of your living room, with the TV off!). No digital devices, no distractions. Talk about your days, your meal, your plans. If you live in a house-share, why not do the same with your flat-mates?

Option D Fairy godmother

- Write a list of the people you appreciate in your life as it is at the moment – they can be those you live with, friends you call or see regularly, colleagues who make your day more enjoyable.
- Pick one of those people who you think deserves a treat, then begin a list of ways you could surprise them. Spend 5 minutes brainstorming.
- It might be that ideas flow easily. If not, try this way of focusing on great treats that don't rely on a huge budget.
- Draw two columns, and in the first, think of ideas for treats that cost money! They're the treats you'd splash out on with a champagne budget.
- In the second column, work out the free or cheap version, for those of us on a lemonade budget. Here are some treats I brainstormed for my partner:

Champagne budget	Lemonade budget
Thai massage at a posh spa (£35)	Foot massage with oils from bathroom cabinet
Movie night at local fancy cinema (£30)	Netflix night – watch the movie he wants (I usually surf the net while he's watching something I don't like) and supply popcorn and cava.
Mexican meal with cocktails (£60)	Buy the ingredients for tacos and cook them together while making cocktails!
Personal training session (£45)	Plan a long bike ride or country walk for the weekend with mini-picnic!

- Now, choose a treat you can offer today or, if not, this week. Enjoy the delight your recipient feels – it's so nice to give out of the blue, without expecting anything in return.

Tip: pets are also eligible for the fairy godmother treatment. A fab long muddy walk with your dog, or 20 minutes playing 'catch the catnip mouse on the end of the stick' with your cat can be mutually rewarding!

5:2 INSPIRATIONS

PET SUBJECTS – THE TRUTH ABOUT CATS AND DOGS

Our four-legged friends are a great boost for our happiness.

Numerous studies show that owning cats or dogs can help lower stress levels, raise self-esteem and reduce any feeling of fearfulness or loneliness.

In one US study, elderly people with pets needed fewer medical appointments than those without them, and in another, a group of HIV-positive men with pets were found to suffer less depressive symptoms than those who didn't own an animal.

On a practical level, dogs also make sure owners stay active, and dog-walkers are a sociable bunch. But even independent-minded cats can encourage human contact – where I live, our cats are always in and out of each other's gardens, and their antics give neighbours plenty to talk about!

Key Activity
feedback

How did the 'reaching out' activity go?

Hopefully your gesture was appreciated. But, as I mentioned above, even the friendliest acts *can* carry a risk of the person on the receiving end not responding exactly as we'd hoped – especially if they see your behaviour as out of character, maybe even suspicious.

So much of the way our relationships work is habitual – and changing any habit takes time and planning. In the Move Week later in the book (page 170, habit-forming for beginners), there's lots of information about replacing bad habits with better ones, but here's a short guide to some of the ways you could identify and reduce flashpoints with your partner, kids, friends or colleagues – and build a better connection instead.

How to break the bickering cycle

It's hard to stop a row once it's started, so prevention is so much better than cure! Of course, it takes two to fix things, and these tips apply to relationships that are basically sound and satisfying, but hit the odd hump in the road. For more serious issues, outside help may be more suitable.

1 **Try to identify the triggers for conflict:**
   - Does it happen at a **particular time of day**? For example, you argue with your children around tea-time, because you're all hungry or snappy – or the rows happen on a Sunday night because everyone's feeling glum about the coming week.
   - Are rows triggered by **a particular behaviour**? For example, your flatmate's habit of always turning the TV to their favourite programme when they get home, even though you're in the middle of watching yours. Or your husband's habit of cutting his toenails while you're in the bath!
   - Do the **causes appear to be trivial**, but are really because you're not facing up to other issues? For example, you argue with your partner when the rubbish needs to be taken out but really you both feel unappreciated/ overburdened.
   - Could a **change in behaviour** be unsettling those close to you? It can confuse others if your behaviour suddenly changes – even for the better – without any apparent reason.

2 **Identify ways to bypass the trigger or cycle**
   Awareness is the first step. Now find solutions. Talking to the others involved can help, so long as you choose a relaxed time to raise the issue.

- If the trigger is a **time of day/week**, change behaviour or timings. For example, move teatime forward, introduce a small snack, avoid discussing homework before everyone's eaten. Or in the Sunday evening example, arrange something fun to do on Sundays to make it a positive time.
- If the **trigger is a behaviour**, discuss the issue in a different room or place and ask the other person for ideas. For example, talk to your flatmate over a coffee in the kitchen about TV viewing hours (and catch-up services online). Or explain to your husband that you like smooth toenails, but romance is lost when you hear the snip of the scissors…
- If the **trigger appears trivial**, explaining what you've observed and asking for comments can help. For example: 'I've noticed that when it comes to rubbish night, we often end up arguing. Is there a way round this?'
- If it's **change that's unsettling others**, explain about *5:2 Your Life*, making it clear that you're doing it to improve your life, not because you're necessarily upset by something they're doing.

3   **Practice makes perfect…**
You only have to watch TV shows like *Supernanny* to know that consistency is the key when it comes to changing behaviour. So do persevere if you see signs of improvements, even if they're not consistent.

4   **But recognise when it's time to get outside help.**
If the conflict is serious and ongoing, and if you ever feel at risk, then seek professional help. It takes two to change – and if your partner ever scares or threatens you, or is unreasonable, then sources of help and support are available – see Part 4: Tools for your 5:2 life on page 352.

Challenge, Connect Day 1
TLC yourself

In this challenge, we're now going to look inwards, connecting with our *own* feelings and needs. Hopefully, by reaching out to others in a kind way, we'll soon be on the receiving end of kindness ourselves. But it can take time for others to begin to do the right thing, so this challenge involves looking after yourself – dishing out some TLC or Tender Loving Care.

There are four options – and I highly recommend Option A, but if you have time, try more than one option.

Option A The Good Things diary

This is quick and easy, but to work best, it's great if you can adopt the habit on all days, not just your 5:2 days. It should only take a few minutes once you're in the swing of it.

You simply aim to jot down some positives at the end of your day (keep your notebook by the bed to remind you to fill it in before you sleep). Aim for:

- three things to feel grateful for each day
- three things you did well.

Don't worry if occasionally you repeat yourself; like any habit, this gets easier. But the positives might include the sunshine or the rainbow you saw, the delicious lunch you had, the great book you're reading or the phone call from a friend. You can also look for silver linings – think of things that appeared to be a cloud but actually made life better: the bus was late, but it meant you walked and saw an advert for a movie you're now planning to see. Or the queue for the supermarket was too long, so you ended up making something delicious from leftovers and saving some money to go out later in the week.

The things you did well can be as basic as you like – it's important to recognise that we make a difference when we do things purposefully, however trivial the tasks seem to be. So it could be the tricky email you sent, the fact you took the stairs instead of the lift, the way you listened to a family member and made them feel better or the great walk you gave the dog!

Option B The me-date/pleasure list revisited

This is about pleasing yourself! And, most important of all, doing it today!

In Discover Week, you had the option of starting your pleasure list, so if you've done that, you have a head start here. Because a me-date is an activity that is all about what *you* find fun. It can be outside, inside, away from the house. The emphasis is less on buying something, more on *experiencing* something.

I adapted this idea from the book *The Artist's Way* by Julia Cameron – she calls them Artist's Dates and they're designed to stimulate creativity. But you don't have to be a would-be artist to enjoy taking some time out to try something different.

So take 5–10 minutes right now to brainstorm a list. Here's mine:

- Go to the new fashion exhibition at local museum.
- Go to Brighton Pavilion (take ID to get resident's discount!).
- Take £5 onto Brighton pier and see what it gets me!
- Open a recipe book I haven't used before, choose a dish and make it today.

- It's a beautiful day – take my phone for a walk and get five shots of rooftops or other things in the big blue sky!

Once you're thinking along these lines, new ideas will occur to you more often, so keep adding to the list. But right now, choose one of these to do either today or this week. If you can't do it today, you're not off the hook.

You must do something for yourself today – or, at the very least, book something today that'll happen this week. Don't postpone – this is important!

Option C Grow your own

The 'making Slough happy' list talks about growing something as being a potential source of happiness – and though it's not an overnight pleasure, there's something fab about planting a seed, or simply nurturing a pot plant from the local florist.

I get the most satisfaction from growing something to eat – so try planting herbs, nurturing a tomato plant or buying a miniature fruit tree. Even if you don't have a garden or window box, anyone can sprout seeds to add to salads; it involves no more equipment than a glass jar, a small piece of fabric, an elastic band and some seeds (it's a bit fiddly but very easy - there's a how-to link in the Resources section, from page 352)!

Option D A great laugh

This is almost effortless but very enjoyable!

What makes *you* laugh?

Whether it's a favourite sitcom, movie, joke book or comic novel, give yourself half an hour to get laughing. My boyfriend cannot resist old episodes of *Only Fools and Horses,* while I'm more of a *Blackadder* or *Alan Partridge* girl. So find that DVD or an episode on YouTube and settle down for some therapeutic laughing.

5:2 MYTH-BUSTING

IS LAUGHTER REALLY THE BEST MEDICINE?

According to several reports, a good laugh can be very beneficial to your health. Can it *really* be that simple? Well, recent studies have suggested that:

- A belly laugh can increase your pain threshold by boosting endorphins (the body's own equivalent of morphine).
- Laughter may also reduce healing time for leg injuries by improving blood flow.
- Regular laughter could help keep the weight off, by acting as NEAT (see Move Week on page 168) and burning energy.

Others have suggested that laughter could even stimulate immune function or improve the results of IVF. Laughter yoga classes – where participants do exercises to stimulate laughter and increase oxygen – can be found in many cities now.

The exact way that laughter might work to produce so many benefits is unclear, but it seems that the harder and longer we laugh, the better the results!

Challenge: feedback
how are you feeling?

So, have you treated yourself to some TLC?

If so, I hope it's put a smile on your face. But what if you're feeling blue?

The flipside of happiness: why sadness isn't always bad news

A lot of this section so far has focused on happiness – how it feels, how we can feel it more often.

But we can't expect to feel deliriously happy all the time.

Research studies have shown that sadness, as well as being an inevitable part of life, is useful for us because it acts as a brake, forcing us to slow down and examine what parts of our lives might not be working, and how we might be able to fix them so we feel better again.

That same research on happiness I outlined earlier (see page 69), suggests that feeling sad for up to 10% of the time can actually be beneficial – because we can learn from feeling lower at times.

But what if your low moments exceed that 10%?

Sadness versus depression

There's a difference between feeling sad, and being depressed.

It's a distinction I am only too familiar with. One of the

reasons I wanted to write this book is that I've experienced depression since my teenage years, and have spent a great deal of time since looking for 'cures'.

I've tried a lot of different things – counselling, medication, exercise, alternative therapies, mindfulness, Cognitive Behavioural Therapy and much more. And then there's the 'self-medication' of drinking or eating too much. I certainly can't claim to have all the answers, but over time I've learned what works for me.

Two things have made the biggest difference: **experience and 5:2 eating.**

Experience has taught me that I *will* feel better in time, and has also provided me with strategies that I know can help me begin to feel less detached and more positive.

5:2 eating has also, quite unexpectedly, proved a huge boost to my mood. Like many of us, I do tend to get grouchy as the summer ends and the days get shorter, but over the last two winters, that hasn't happened. In fact, as I've maintained my weekly fasting I've found my energy levels rose higher and my mood was buoyant.

I later read research suggesting that intermittent fasting – the technical name for 5:2 – can alter brain chemistry and boost mood very effectively. iIt's a complex area, but there is interesting research into how chemical changes to the brain may raise mood. My own experience has certainly been very positive but we need to be cautious, of course.

5:2 isn't a 'cure' – and though many on our forums have reported mood-boosting effects, others haven't. But it's a strategy worth trying. 5:2 has also helped me see the wood for the trees. The focus on small achievements, and on taking control of things in manageable ways, has been one of the most enlightening, liberating approaches to making things better that I've ever come across (and I have owned a *lot* of self-help books over the years).

Time to seek help?

If things feel bleak day after day, then you need to seek help – depression isn't something you should handle alone.

It's important to recognise when professional medical advice is the best option to take. I'm not ashamed of having taken medication for depression – sadly, it doesn't work for everyone, but I've had positive effects from it, helping to cushion some of life's blows while I work on other practical solutions. The strategies in this book can be excellent but you often do need to feel quite robust before you begin to tackle some of them.

I also know that 'connecting' with other people can be the hardest thing if you're suffering from the blues. It's the isolation of depression that is often the most difficult part – that sense of being separated from the highs and the good things in life. People often describe it as watching the world through glass, or gauze, but not being able to cross over and take part.

For many of us, the smallest steps – meeting a friend for coffee or taking a walk through the park – can begin to make a difference even if, at first, it feels a little like going through the motions.

The online self-assessment questionnaire on the British NHS website – nhs.uk/Tools/Pages/depression.aspx – can help you discover what to do next if you're concerned about your own mood or if you feel that sadness is lasting longer than usual or proving disabling.

Your first port of call is your GP/family doctor, who can point you in the right direction, and discuss whether professional counselling or medication is an option.

Alongside professional help, there are practical tools you can use – both online, and offline. The NHS often uses Cognitive Behavioural Therapy as a strategy for anxiety, compulsive behaviours and depression – read more at nhs.uk/conditions/cognitive-behavioural-therapy/Pages/Introduction.aspx.

You can also monitor your mood – and what factors affect it positively or negatively – using apps. Moodscope.com is an interesting one: a website and app that uses an innovative 'playing card' scoring system; while MoodPanda.com has a quicker, simpler interface. Or try charting your menstrual cycles (or those of someone close to you!) to see what effect that has on your mood. None of these are a substitute for medical help but they can help you to identify patterns and solutions.

But it doesn't take the latest technology to help you feel better. Sometimes, going back to basics is the best way forward.

5:2 INSPIRATIONS

WRITING WRONGS

You already own one of the most powerful tools for deepening your understanding of your life, any difficult experiences, and how your mind works.

It's called a pen.

Expressive writing – the act of writing about traumatic or difficult events – can improve your mood and general health. Pioneering research in the 1980s by Dr James Pennebaker, former Chair of Psychology at the University of Texas, showed benefits including fewer visits to the doctor, a strengthening of the immune system and better psychological health.

Pennebaker's theory is that if we've 'buried' traumas in our past, then it stresses the body, physically and mentally – so, allowing those feelings to come out through writing then reduces that stress. His work has been repeated several hundred times all over the world, with similar results.

Today's Bonus Activity involves trying out this technique if *you* feel there may be past experiences or memories that might still be holding you back.

Bonus Activity, Connect Day 1:
the write way

A word of warning: if you are very low at the moment, or receiving treatment for depression, do please check with your doctor or therapist before trying this.

Guidelines for expressive writing

Expressive writing is simple. It involves writing about your feelings for 15 minutes.

I'll admit this is one of those times when you may want to

try the activity more frequently than twice during the week. Studies into the effectiveness of expressive writing have involved people writing each day for at least three or four consecutive days rather than twice a week. So, if you can set aside that time, you may see quicker results.

You also need to find a time in your day to write – Pennebaker's guidelines suggest writing at the end of the working day, or before bedtime.

- What you write is your business – this is never going to be seen by anyone else.
- Topics might include:
  - what is worrying you right now – difficult decisions, dreams, struggles in relationships or with addictions
  - difficult experiences in the past – especially anything you've been avoiding thinking about or talking about for any period
  - anything you feel is affecting you in an unhealthy way.
- **You can write however you like** – with pen and paper, or using a computer. You can even dictate into a recorder if you can't write.
- **Don't worry about *what* you're writing – grammar and spelling really don't matter**. If you find yourself writing about the same thing – or even repeating the same words – **just keep going for the full 15 minutes.**
- **You can write about the same topic each day, or something different.**
- **Many participants do find it upsetting,** with some crying during the process, and others feeling down afterwards. But studies suggest most feel better after a couple of hours.

- **If you find a particular topic too upsetting, switch to something else: you don't have to push yourself further than you feel able to go.**

When you've finished:
- You can re-read what you've written if you like – either before starting on subsequent days, or at the end.
- Or you can simply throw the writing away or destroy it: by burning, tearing up the paper, or throwing it into the sea.
- Review how you feel after you've finished your four days. Keep going if you like. Or simply see how you feel in a couple of weeks. Do you feel that the writing has helped?

If you want to read more from Pennebaker himself, or watch a video, there are links in the resources section from page 352.

Ending Day 1 on a high

Our main focus on this first day has been making ourselves, and the people close to us, feel good – and taking the time to notice and enjoy the nicer things about life.

I definitely recommend keeping your Good Things diary (see page 79 to remind you of what it involves) between now and your next 5:2 day – and adding to your pleasure and me-dates list .

On Connect Day 2, we'll be looking more at how we can make the most of the world and community we live in.

CONNECT DAY 2

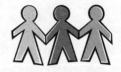

Welcome back!

Have you made the time to 'TLC' yourself *and* to do something good for someone you care about – and that there's been a positive outcome. Maybe something to write in your Good Things diary? And if you're trying out expressive writing, I hope you're finding it enlightening.

Today, we're broadening our outlook. Connecting isn't just about improving relationships with people in our immediate circle, it's also about our place in the world.

The street where you live

As kids, we often used to write our addresses like this:

Kate Harrison
1a Smile Street
Happytown
Cheeryshire
England
Great Britain
United Kingdom
Europe
The world
The solar system
The universe…

But once we're adults, and busy or stressed, our world often shrinks till we struggle to see beyond the walls of our house, or the fabric 'walls' of our office cubicle.

This week is about widening our perspective again and appreciating what's around us.

It might sound a bit hippy-dippy – but there is good evidence that connecting with where we live and our surroundings will make us happier.

Remember the research from Connect Day 1 about how being engaged in politics is one of the factors in people feeling happier?

Having common interests and goals, whether they're political or social, makes us feel better about ourselves and others. On the flip side, if we feel threatened where we live, or disconnected from our neighbours, our isolation increases.

Neighbours, everybody needs good neighbours!

I was addicted to *Neighbours* on TV as a teenager. Though it was pretty debatable whether the folks in Ramsay Street counted as good neighbours, what with all the gossip and carrying on!

As a kid, we moved house a lot, and I've continued that trend as an adult, moving to seven different cities. I've lived in leafy suburbs and city centres – my personal preference is to be as central as possible, because I don't like driving and I do like to be close to 'life'.

But you can feel *too* close – in London, my flat was two doors down from a crack house. Yet that bothered me less than the isolation. My neighbours moved very regularly so it was hard to get to know anyone.

When I moved into my boyfriend's rental flat in a leafier area, the development was brand new, overlooking the river. But the security gates and lack of communal space meant we saw our neighbours for the first time on the day we moved out, when one complained we were hogging the lift with our boxes!

I love where we live now, in a Victorian cottage in the centre of Brighton. Yes, it can be noisy at times, but there's a real sense of community, with street parties and lots of chat on the doorsteps. What's interesting is that it hasn't always been like that – locals say that there's more community spirit now than forty years ago. Never mind fretting about the good old days – it is possible to find neighbourliness whenever and wherever you are.

We're lucky to have found an area that suits us – it wouldn't suit everyone (the car parking is a nightmare, our yard is tiny and the drunks have been known to use our garden wall as a loo!) but it has what *we* need.

Of course, if your neighbours are truly unbearable, there is help available – see Part 4: Tools for your 5:2 life. But for today's first activity, we're going to focus on loving your area more…

Key Activity, Connect Day 2
local love

It's time to discover what your patch has to offer! Pick one, or more, of these three options. They should all give you a warmer feeling about your community without too much effort.

Option A Do local

Find out what events are happening in your local area – and buy a ticket for an event coming up. Good sources of information are your local paper or their website, the council website, your local library or community centre information board or the window of your local shop.

It might be a concert, an amateur drama production, a laughter yoga course (see the challenge from Connect Day 1 for a reminder about the positive effects laughter can have), an historical walk or a new class. September, January and after Easter are the best times to find new courses at local schools and colleges.

Bonus points for: something involving singing or music! Research shows that being a member of a choir or country dancing class can boost your mood.

Option B Buy/eat local

For one day – preferably today if you can – only buy or consume products that come from your local area or county. Buy in local shops, ask where the fruit or veg comes from, find a bakery where they bake their own bread. Or go to the pub and enjoy a pint from a local brewery!

If you live in a small town or village and the choice isn't as wide, then investigate signing up for a fruit and veg box service from local farmers or find the nearest farm shop.

You could also look up a local, traditional recipe and try it out. Sussex Pond Pudding, here I come!

Bonus points for: sharing your local produce with your next-door neighbour!

Option C See local

Take your camera or smartphone out for a walk – and leave your MP3 player at home. Look around for things to photograph that you haven't noticed before. You can often find guides to local walks or sites online, or even a guided walk to download (in which case you are allowed to take the MP3 player!).

Drop in on a café or shop you've never visited on the way home.

Bonus points for: posting a photo on your Facebook or Twitter account explaining what you love about your area!

Key Activity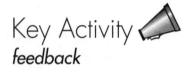
feedback

How did that go?

We often take where we live for granted, getting into the same routines and taking the same routes. Like many of the other activities in this book, this part is simply about taking a fresh look. Often we only go to our area's most famous or beautiful places when we have visitors – but why wait? Seeing the place through a visitor's eyes can help you remember why you like where you live!

Hopefully you've also found new ideas, foods, or places to experience: and if you're keeping a Good Things Diary, this activity could feature!

The bigger picture: what are we here for?

Questions don't get much bigger than this… and finding the answer can take a lifetime. In the meantime, small acts of kindness or generosity can help us feel better about our place in the world.

Of course, if you have a sense of faith or spirituality, then that may provide you with answers to the 'what are we here for' question. I'm not a religious person, but my central belief in life is that we should do as we would be done by, i.e. treat others the way we want to be treated ourselves. I don't always manage it, but I think that reaching out and offering help to others is one very practical way to stop a cycle of negative or self-centred thoughts.

If that sounds a bit worthy, it doesn't have to be. We can't all commit to volunteering regularly, for example, or to trekking across mountain ranges to raise funds for charity. But we can find ways to do things that we'll enjoy and will also make us feel more connected to the communities we belong to – whether the communities are based on geography, shared beliefs or a personal passion!

Because passion can be as important as proximity in the digital age.

Community spirit

You can't always choose your neighbours, but your virtual neighbours can offer an alternative to the cup of sugar over the garden fence. Online communities can offer that sense of being part of something bigger.

Our 5:2 Facebook group is one example – it's grown from six members to 20,000+ – and though there's the odd squabble, the mutual support has made a huge difference to people's successes. Plus, it allows us to debate the minutiae of our diets in the kind of detail that would bore our families or work colleagues to tears.

On a larger scale, look at the growth of the UK-based site, Mumsnet – one of the most successful online communities ever. The community has members from all locations and backgrounds with parenthood in common. Yet the discussions have moved way, way beyond debating the best ways to survive potty-training or the terrible twos. The friendships and connections are now life-changing. And Mumsnet also has a huge effect on the national debate.

Even tools like Twitter – often criticised for inciting arguments or threatening behaviour – can create community spirit. The response to rioting across the UK in the summer of 2011 was striking, as neighbours came together via Tweets to help clear up the areas. And on an international level, social networking is used to highlight and campaign against war crimes and human rights abuses and even co-ordinate protests.

Finding your community is much easier than it used to be – and can make it simple to find ways to make a difference.

Challenge, Connect Day 2
community spirit

There are six options, all designed to make getting involved enjoyable and straightforward.

Option A Down with the kids

Option B Be neighbourly

Option C Sign up to a cause

Option D Donate money or items to a local charity

Option E Donate time

Option F Learn first aid basics

Choose the one that appeals to you – and make firm plans either to do the challenge today or within the next few days.

Option A Down with the kids

What do your children think matters most in their lives? What do they like or worry about when it comes to the world – and area – they live in?

If you don't know, ask them – and then help them do something about it. Whether it's making jewellery from recycled materials, or inventing a way to fund-raise for endangered species (for example by being sponsored to do something – most charities have plenty of ideas on their website), make it something fun you can do together.

It could even be something as simple as heading down to the nearest skate park or basketball park and taking some pictures to upload to a community site or Facebook page.

Option B Be neighbourly

Invite a neighbour around for a cup of tea, or offer them something from your garden or a slice of home-made cake.

It's often hard to make the first move if you've been living somewhere for a while, so sharing something personal can really break the ice.

Option C Sign up to a cause

What *really* bothers you about how the world works? Remember the causes you were passionate about when you were a teenager? In my case, it was equality and justice, but paying the bills has become too much of a preoccupation these days.

Luckily, having your voice heard is much easier now: if you're in the UK, then epetitions.direct.gov.uk offers the chance to browse the latest campaigns and add your support. The Australian equivalent, gopetition.com.au, has a range of international, national and local campaigns featured.

As an aside, when I was editing this book, my fantastic colleague Peta told me about her experience on an e-petitions site. She'd gone online to sign up for a worthy cause… but was drawn to a petition to make the 1980s song *Gold* by Spandau Ballet the new British national anthem!

She signed on the spot.

As this petition was launched in 2007, and as yet the British anthem is still *God Save the Queen,* you could conclude e-petitions are a waste of time, or a joke. Yet Peta said signing the petition made her feel really happy and light-hearted for a long time afterwards – at the idea, but also at the fact that she was part of a 'community' who could engage in that kind of silly but quite charming campaign.

So – what will *you* change? Either go online and find three causes that you feel strongly about – or choose one you feel very strongly about and write to your MP or to someone else you believe can change things. The writetothem.com website makes it easy to contact your MP in the UK.

Option D Donate money or items to a local charity

If you have money or items to spare, they can make a big difference. Start a bag of charity items and keep it somewhere hand. Then, when it's full, take it to your local charity shop.

If you can afford it, charities also appreciate financial donations – a good way to find a cause you'd like to support is via justgiving.com or localgiving.com for local causes.

You can also decide to support charities by direct debit or just keeping your eyes open – many animal welfare charities have a box at the local supermarket and ask you to buy an extra tin of food and leave it on the way out.

The UK's foodbank network is also growing all the time (on the 5:2 Facebook page, we raised £1,000 for them by donating the cost of a sandwich or a pound for each pound we'd lost in weight) and you can donate to them financially or take along food donations to make a difference to those who need it. Search for your nearest bank at trusselltrust.org/map

In Australia, foodbank.org.au offered almost 31 million meals to those who needed them in 2012.

Option E Donate time

Volunteering doesn't have to involve a regular commitment if that doesn't suit you – charities are now much more flexible in the way that volunteers can work with them.

A good place to begin is do-it.org where you can find local charities or national causes which may need help for targeted fund-raising weeks or events. Or look into mentoring or workplace volunteering via sites like Timebank.org.uk

Alternatively, look at running your own event – it's very easy via sites like justgiving.com in the UK. Or take part in a national day, like Macmillan's World's Biggest Coffee Morning, or Breast Cancer Care's Strawberry Tea in the UK, or a Girls' Night In or Pink Ribbon event in aid of cancer charities in Australia.

Option F Learn first aid basics

I recently discovered first-hand how vital first aid training can be, and am incredibly grateful that I had the chance to attend a course at work years ago. Even though my skills were rusty, the course prepared me mentally for a moment where every second counted.

You can sign up to take a course locally – Google is the best source of local providers – but in the meantime, even watching a video about the basics of hands-only Cardio-Pulmonary Resuscitation could give you enough knowledge to save a life. I particularly recommend life-saver.org.uk which is an interactive film/game which takes you through realistic scenarios where you learn how you could help.

Challenge: feedback

Whatever you've done, or signed up to do, I hope it's shown you how simple it can be to get involved. And, potentially, how rewarding.

The more you tune into your local area, or the global issues you care about, the more you're likely to notice ways to get involved (see the Puppy Effect on page 58).

Connecting online

If that's whetted your appetite, try some of these sites that will help you make more community connections:

csv.org.uk runs the Make a Difference Campaign every October and specializes in mentoring, too.

yoursquaremile.co.uk – I love this site. Just type in your postcode and it allows you to share ideas, find local charities, organise community events and even report annoyances via fixmystreet.com.

projectaustralia.org.au is a not-for-profit organisation that helps you start, or get involved in, community projects.

freecycle.org – The Freecycle Network operates globally to help local groups (moderated by local volunteers) find new homes and uses for our goods, to keep good stuff out of landfills.

Finally, today's optional Bonus Activity brings together all your research and hard work to create a guide that'll keep helping you to love where you live.

Bonus Activity, Connect Day 2
Your Personal Yellow Pages

As the internet has grown, the good old Yellow Pages directory has shrunk, or even disappeared. Most of the contents of that encyclopaedia-sized book have gone online.

So we're going to make a replacement – but instead of being bulked out with services you never use, your *personal* directory of local highlights will be something you can use and grow all the time.

The idea is to create a scrapbook or online directory of the places you love, the events you'd like to take part in and even the best shops or services. You can use it for inspiration when you're looking for something to do or somewhere to go.

- For a physical 'book, **choose a scrapbook or display book** (with the see-through pockets for leaflets).
- OR for a virtual version, **use a Facebook page or a Pinterest.com board**, or even set up a blog to share what you're creating. The app **Evernote.com** would also work well for this as it allows you to clip pictures and text. You could also create a personal map on **Google Maps** where you can include favourite walks, sights and places to eat.
- Think of **two or three headings** to begin with. Here are some suggestions:
    - Food and drink
    - Great outdoors
    - Favourite walks or bike rides
    - Entertainment
    - Annual events
    - Sports venues
    - Essential contacts – not just the police or hospital but also plumbers, electricians and hairdressers you trust and like
    - History
    - Best buildings
    - Most photogenic or famous people!
- Begin to **compile your entries** – use business cards, photos and pictures as well as numbers.
- **Do be aware of privacy settings if you are compiling a directory online** – if you're making it public, be wary of

identifying yourself by name or address. Or choose to be the only user to see your notes.

- **Keep adding to your guide:** it's great to keep it up to date, and a good resource when you need something to do, or even when you have a problem to address.

Connect Week: key points

Here's a summary of our key points from this week:

- Feeling connected is one of the keys to feeling more satisfied about life.
- Make firm plans to do things with friends and family, and to reconnect with people around you: it may feel awkward at first but will soon become a good habit.
- Feelings of sadness can help us understand what's wrong with our lives – but if your low mood lasts for a long time or is affecting your life, always see your doctor.
- Recording how you feel and positive things in your life can raise your mood…
- … while spending time writing about the things that concern you can help lower your stress levels and have other benefits.
- Communities of like-minded people aren't always geographical – you can make connections online more easily than ever.

Week 3

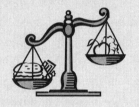

Simplicity is the ultimate sophistication.

Leonardo da Vinci

Week 3: checking in

How are you doing this week? Did you find the Connect activities helpful or revealing? Let's quickly review how it went.

- Are you noticing more about what's going on around you in your local community? Keep an eye out as you walk or commute, or take photos on your phone of posters or flyers for events you'd like to try.

- Have you been trying out the Good Things Diary or expressive writing? These may bring instant results, or take a little longer to have an effect, but both have made a big difference to people's lives.

- My experience: I recently spent quite a lot of time in our local hospital and it's made me feel part of my community in a whole new way. I was humbled by the humanity of the medical staff. I also realised that when the time is right, I want to contribute, whether it's through fund-raising, writing to the health trust to say thanks or simply dropping off the magazines I've read rather than recycling them. Or possibly doing all three!

Simplify

THIS WEEK'S AIM:
to clear unnecessary clutter – mental, physical and financial –
and enjoy the space it creates to live better.

Introduction

We're on a mission to declutter your life this week – but if you think that means living in a cold minimalist home, with none of your favourite things, then don't worry – by the time we've finished, the things you value will be centre stage so you can enjoy them even more.

On Day 1, we'll focus on simplifying your surroundings and the things you do every day – so you can see the wood for the trees.

And on Day 2 we'll look at financial clutter – so you can begin to feel more in control of money, rather than letting it control you.

It's all about making the very best of what we have and building on what makes us happy.

SIMPLIFY QUIZ

Let's start with three quick, light-hearted questions about your life.

This week: **how your life works**

1　How would you feel about someone having a nose in your kitchen cupboards?

    A   Deeply ashamed – the cupboards are in a terrible mess, and I'd be worried they might injure themselves on a falling baked bean tin.

    B   OK – I don't think they're the best organised spaces in the house, but they're no worse than anyone else's and I know where everything is!

    C   Proud – I love to be organised and my cupboards are a thing of beauty.

    D   Pleased – so long as they also agreed to give them a good tidy up. I never get the time. An archaeologist might also find some prehistoric pasta in there too.

2　Do you know how much is in your bank account right now?

    A   No. I'm scared to look.

    B   Roughly. I check a couple of times a week.

    C   Down to the last penny.

    D   I know how much *isn't* in there – but I've got an agreed overdraft and it helps cushion me. No one I know who is any fun has money in the bank.

3　How do you feel about delegating tasks like cleaning, washing, finances?

    A   It's a good idea in principle, but I wouldn't want to delegate anything right now because it would reveal what a mess I'm in.

    B   I already share tasks with other people in the house and would love a cleaner if I could afford one.

C   No! If a job's worth doing, it's worth doing yourself.
    Plus, I'd hate all my systems to be disrupted!
D   Bring it on. I'd delegate getting up in the morning if
    I could.

If you found yourself drawn to…

Mostly As: chances are your life, home or finances feel out of control right now. But there is hope – by the end of your two 5:2 days, you can get yourself back on track!

Mostly Bs: you're getting there, but could do with being a bit more organised. There are lots of tips to help you save time to do the things you enjoy more.

Mostly Cs: you are an organisational superstar – but being a perfectionist about everything can be stressful. This week will help you work out where to stay in control, and where you might be able to afford to relax a little…

Mostly Ds: There's nothing wrong with being laid back about some things, but by focusing on a few key concerns, you could afford to be even more chilled out.

SIMPLIFY DAY 1

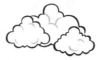

Give me shelter

What are the absolute basics that we need to survive?

Why not spend a couple of minutes thinking about *your* answers? Keep it to the very minimum. My list would include food, water, air and shelter from the elements.

I am cheating slightly because I've just looked up Maslow's Hierarchy of Needs. It sounds very technical but is, at heart, a list of what a psychologist, Abraham Maslow, believed were the basic human needs and motivations. He saw those needs as being pyramid shaped, with his own list of basic human priorities at the bottom – he thought we'd only progress to the higher needs once we'd secured the fundamentals.

You don't need to study it in detail, but so many of these needs are addressed in this book: friends, family and respect in the Connect chapter; health in the Eating Plan and Move chapters; employment and achievement in Do! But in this section we're looking at money and shelter: or, in other words, the roof over your head.

'Security' is about more than staying warm or dry in bad weather, or being shaded from fierce sunlight. It's about a retreat, a place that allows us to be ourselves, that energises us and reminds us of what we love about life.

Yet how many of us can really say that's true?

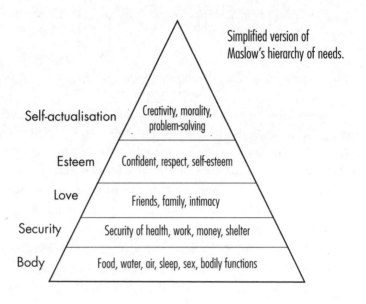

Simplified version of Maslow's hierarchy of needs.

Self-actualisation — Creativity, morality, problem-solving

Esteem — Confident, respect, self-esteem

Love — Friends, family, intimacy

Security — Security of health, work, money, shelter

Body — Food, water, air, sleep, sex, bodily functions

Ideal home?

Most of us don't have the 'ideal home'. Yours might suffer from:

- mess/dirt
- poor state of repair/lack of light
- lack of space
- too much clutter
- lack of security.

Right now, there seem to be many TV shows and newspaper pieces about extreme hoarders or infestations of pests. But even the mildest case of clutter or lack of space can affect your quality of life.

And even the items that supposedly make our lives easier can sometimes seem to conspire against us… take technology, for example.

The case for the prosecution: the charger drawer

Ten years ago, I didn't need a drawer just to store leads and connectors and plugs.

Now I do, and it's getting more and more like a giant mound of black spaghetti. Trying to find the lead I need to recharge my toothbrush or camera turns into a highly frustrating 10-minute job. It's a trivial example of the way modern life can complicate things and rob us of time, rather than simplify things and save time.

The case for the defence: the e-book

But the physical space taken up by chargers has been saved by another bit of technology – the e-book.

As an avid reader, I find it incredibly hard to get rid of books… and my shelves are bowing under the pressure. I was sceptical about e-readers, but I tried a Kindle and haven't looked back. My shelves are still standing, and it's also made holidays so much less back-breaking (I am a very fast reader, so used to pack seven books for a week-long holiday). I still buy physical books too, but it's an example of a technology that really works for me (though I still struggle to find the charger).

The verdict

It's all about working out how to control our gadgets, not let them control us. And, of course, the same applies to our homes generally. The more disorganised and cluttered your home, the harder it is to live 'efficiently'. In a moment, we're going to improve *your* space, but first, an inspiring example of how the right surroundings can change not just your home, but your behaviour too.

5:2 INSPIRATIONS

THE SHED EFFECT

This is the story of how a shed can change your life. Author Nicola Morgan – who writes novels and non-fiction like *Blame My Brain*, about teen behaviour – credits her shed with revolutionising her working life. But even if you don't have a shed, you can learn from her experience.

Like many people who work from home (and many of us in offices too!), Nicola had gradually fallen into a pattern that wasn't good for her *or* her productivity:

I got the work done – never missed a deadline yet – but it felt unhappily ill-disciplined, ineffective, pathetic. Not so much work–life balance, as collapsed in a heap of tangled intentions.

But in May 2011, everything changed. How? Nicola got a shed in her garden, and relocated her workspace... instantly, she became more efficient and enjoyed her work more.

Nicola mentioned her experience to a psychologist friend who identified what had happened as something known as **stimulus generalisation**.

The idea is that our environment and 'stimuli' – whatever is going on around us, including sounds, sights, smells and routines – reinforce the behaviours that are familiar, including bad habits.

If you've ever wanted to cut down on smoking or drinking, you might identify with this – certain times of day or social settings are more likely to trigger the behaviour you want to change. But it also means you can **manipulate your surroundings** to improve your chances of success.

In Nicola's case, the change was to her daily routine.

Effectively, I had suddenly changed almost all the stimuli around me, in one go. This made my existing desire to change working habits much easier; it enabled an immediate fresh slate, allowing new stimuli to create new habits. In the same way, an addict is encouraged, as part of therapy, to remove all physical aspects of the situations in which previously he took the addictive substance.

If you'd like more detail about the transformation, Nicola has written a blog post about it – see the link in the Resources section from page 352 – with suggestions for other home workers, including:

- changing the room where you work, or moving your furniture/changing your view
- redecorating or buying new furniture
- changing your working hours or taking a briefcase to work, even if 'work' is simply in the next room.

But it can work for anyone. My partner works in the management side of the construction industry, a very different kind of job to a stay-at-home writer, but he adapted the suggestions: moved his desk, brought in a radio to mask distracting noises, changed the picture on his computer desktop. He even decided to change what he wore to work, wearing a tie more often, even though his colleagues often dressed down.

No shed required, but he reckoned it transformed his working day.

In today's key activity, we're not actively setting out to change bad habits – simply change a small area of your home. But that fresh start could trigger more exciting changes. Later, in today's challenge, we'll be looking more at the link between environment and behaviour.

Key Activity, Simplify Day 1
the *sensational* makeover

Are you ready for a room makeover?

And before you worry about a 1990s *Changing Rooms* style revamp, complete with gold lamé bedspread and oxblood red feature walls, there is no fancy designer involved in this process (unless you're a fancy interior designer yourself).

In keeping with all our 5:2 principles, this is about making small changes to create a big difference. No one can sort their entire home out in half an hour, but this task will make an immediate difference. It focuses on the senses, to create a *sensational* makeover.

Step 1

- Set a timer for 20 minutes. Pick a room in your home that frustrates you or stresses you out (I'm not including kids' bedrooms here; choose somewhere you personally spend time). Even if you're tidy, there's probably an area that could be working better. Or you could apply this to your space at work.
- Take your notebook into the room so you are on site to deal with the problem!
- Start by listing the problems, and divide your page into three columns to help you find solutions too:

Problem	Quick/free solution	Needs more time/money

Step 2

- Now you're going to brainstorm ideas to make things better. Because we often can't see the wood for the trees when we're in a familiar space, we're going to use the five senses to identify what you can improve.

Sense 1: sight

- What looks right and what looks wrong in the room? What winds you up most about the space and how could you deal with it?
- Take a good look – there may be things you've got so used to that you don't notice that really don't belong.

For example, my choice of room is my spare bedroom/office and I notice:

- big piles of paperwork about to topple over
- two ugly printers dominating the space
- what the hell is that plastic washing tub doing on top of the wardrobe?
- Now list the problems and brainstorm different solutions. Don't rule anything out at this stage – sometimes the wildest solutions are the best. See the table below for examples.

Problem	Quick/free solution	Needs more time/ money
Big piles of paper-work.	Make an 'urgent' pile and put the rest in the cupboard. Find a folder to put the urgent stuff into. Burn/recycle it all!	Put aside an hour this weekend to deal with urgent stuff. Put aside more time next week to deal with the less urgent stuff. Dump all the non-urgent stuff in the recycling?!

Ugly printer.	Move furniture so I can't see printer when I work.	Cover it with stickers? Paint it? Buy a newer, more compact printer or find a cupboard to put it in? Do I really need two printers? Give one away on Freecycle?
Plastic tub	Put it in the kitchen or shed! Solved!	

Now work your way through the other senses. (Don't worry, they probably won't be as lengthy.)

Sense 2: hearing

- Is this room noisy?
  - You can't always control external noise but internal noise can be masked or improved.
  - Something as simple as swapping talk radio for music can make a difference – I am a big fan of a cheesy '80s station when I am working, as it isn't as distracting as talk radio.
  - If you have a budget, noise-cancelling headphones can be worth investigating – or ear plugs are a cheap and cheerful option!

Sense 3: smell

- Smelly, stuffy rooms are uninspiring.
  - Make the most of fresh air! Open your windows at least once a day to let stuffiness out and air in.
  - A few aromatherapy oils in a burner or just dripped onto ceramic light bulb rings can inspire or relax. Lavender is perfect for relaxation, rose geranium lifts the

mood, and zesty scents like mandarin or lime are great for concentration.

- Or make it even easier with room sprays or candles – but do sniff before buying, as they vary in how nice (or nasty) they are.

Sense 4: touch

- Threadbare carpets or scratchy bedding can make a place feel neglected, while cold bathroom or kitchen floor tiles can be miserable in winter.
  - Homeware stores like IKEA stock rugs or bedding for all budgets…
  - A pair of fluffy slippers can be a budget option so your feet needn't suffer!
  - A soft blanket or funky cushion can make a difference to how welcoming a room feels. Even a functional room like a bathroom or home office can be improved with fluffy towels or a cushion on the office chair (though I think cushions divide the world along gender lines – my boyfriend hates them with a passion).

Sense 5: taste

- Your personal taste makes your home come to life: the things you use, the colours you like and the objects that mean something to you are so important.
  - Adding even a single object that reflects your personal taste can make a place more welcoming. I love second-hand shops for random pieces of glassware or unusual ceramics. Freecycle can also help with larger items like bookshelves or wardrobes.

- If you don't have room for big items, even a new mug or coaster or photo on the mantelpiece can make you smile.

Step 3

- Take 5 minutes to identify three or four solutions from your entire sense survey. Choose the ones that will make the biggest difference, with a mix of free, fast solutions and longer-term ones.
- **Pick one of the solutions and do it now** – and schedule the others with firm time frames – use your online calendar or diary to schedule reminders. You could:
  - clear piles of things away into bags or cupboards (and schedule a time to tackle them properly)
  - join your local Freecycle and add an appeal for something you need, or an offer for something you want to give away
  - open the window and light an aromatherapy burner
  - find an old radio, tune it to a favourite station and have a celebration dance!

How was that for you?

Even if you're a fabulously organised person, I hope the makeover gave you some practical ideas to improve your environment and your day-to-day life. Like Nicola and her shed, your revamped space could give you a whole new perspective on life, too.

Challenge, Simplify Day 1
the delegator

For our challenge, we're going to focus on household jobs that need to be done but you'd really rather not tackle. There's an advert for a household cleaning product which ends with the line: *loves the jobs you hate*. The idea is that it's strong enough to tackle the grimiest cleaning jobs.

But what if you could do that for much more than a stained sink? What if you could pass on your most hated jobs, for good?

That's what our challenge today is about: finding more time to focus on the things you want to do, by eliminating or finding ways around the things you don't like doing. It's like being Arnie in *The Terminator,* except that instead of, um, terminating – you're delegating.

Don't assume you have to pay out to get jobs done. Yes, some *might* involve money… but then again it may be about swapping duties with a family member or a neighbour. Or even finding a techie way to delegate.

Step 1

List all the jobs you avoid or hate. Then score your hate level out of 10 – with 10 as the most hated, and 0 as 'actually I don't hate it that much after all'.

I asked my Facebook friends which jobs they'd love to delegate:

- **Housework**: tidying, cleaning, especially loo cleaning, cat litter tray cleaning and potty emptying, recycling, putting bins out, oven cleaning, hoovering, defrosting the freezer.

- **Laundry/Washing**: hanging out washing/getting it in, ironing (lots loathe that one), washing and drying up (lots of people like one and hate the other), un-stacking the dishwasher, pairing socks.
- **Cooking**: grocery shopping, cooking generally, planning the week's meals, ordering takeaways (Clare has to write the dishes down because otherwise she'll get it wrong), making breakfast (Imogen would love someone to prepare her a fresh fruit salad every morning).
- **Household management**: paying bills, getting things repaired, finding workmen, complaining, phoning call centres, present and card shopping, organising holidays, sorting out doctor/dentist appointments (Jude called it being a 'Ghostbuster' – who you gonna call?), car stuff, going to the post office, gardening, DIY, *remembering everything!*
- **Kids' stuff**: doing their homework, chauffeuring, clearing up after them!
- **Work stuff**: filing, bookkeeping, tax returns, social media for a business
- **Big financial decisions**: pensions, insurance, moving accounts, making money, worrying about finances!

Step 2

Now pick your most hated jobs and brainstorm ways you could delegate them.

For example:

- Swap Delegation (SD) – is there someone in your household or neighbourhood who might not hate the task, and could trade with a task you're happy to do?

- Benefits In Kind Delegation (BIKD) – do you have kids looking to earn pocket money – or a partner or housemate who'd take on your loathed job in return for benefits in kind, like being cooked a nice meal or… well, I'll let you work out what might motivate those closest to you.
- Passive-Aggressive Delegation (PAD) – tell others you're not going to do the job anymore and make it their responsibility – if you can handle the mess…
- Technological Delegation (TD) – is there an app, software or service that could make life easier and reduce the time spent on the tasks you loathe?
- Paid Delegation (PD) – cleaning or ironing services are the most obvious, but you can get help from concierge or 'wife for hire' services to do the most mundane jobs now.
- 'Just Say No' (JSN) – are there any jobs you can simply stop doing? Or do far less frequently without ill-effects? A milder version is 'Just Say Sometimes' (JSS).
- Share The Load (STL) – can you share duties with people with similar responsibilities or needs?
- Simple Appeal (SA) – appeal to the better nature of those around you. Explain you're struggling and would appreciate some help!

I've put together a few examples.

Job	Hate score	Delegation ideas
Organising presents/cards	8/10	Declare a moratorium on gifts and cards, explaining you don't expect them from people anymore and won't give them either! (JSN) Send e-cards and vouchers instead (TD) Sign up for a card service that will remind you of occasions coming up and even send cards on your behalf (TD/PD)
Ironing	10/10	Use an ironing service (PD) Stop ironing: many things – shirts are the exception – are fine if you pull them into shape before line-drying them. And definitely stop ironing knickers, socks or tea towels! (JSN) Find a housemate or neighbour who loves ironing (yes, those people do exist) and offer to do something they hate in return (SD)
Dog walking in the dark	9/10	Hire a dog-walker (PD) Draw up a rota with dog-owning neighbours to do the after-dark walks – or you do the morning walk, they do the evening (STL) Make the morning walk much longer so the dog is more exhausted and needs a shorter walk in the evening! (JSS)

Challenge: feedback

How did that go? Some of the delegation ideas might seem flippant but the best solutions sometimes come from the unexpected.

On day 2 we'll be focusing on finances. Don't groan, I promise it'll be a positive experience. To prepare for that, today's bonus activity involves thinking about how little money it can take to brighten our mood.

Bonus Activity, Simplify Day 1: the element of surprise

What's the price of feeling happier? It could be smaller than you think…

There's a German study by psychologist Norbert Schwarz which shows that less than 10p – or a dime, 10 cents – can have a dramatic effect on your outlook. It's not the amount – it's the unexpectedness that makes the difference.

Schwarz left a low-value coin – less than 10p – on top of a photocopier for users to find. Later, he interviewed people about how satisfied they felt with their lives, and those who'd found the coin rated their satisfaction levels higher than those who didn't – though they didn't make any connection between the very small stroke of luck and their mood.

For this bonus activity, we're going to build on the work of the Good Things Diary from the Connect Week. But we're going to go further and actively look for ways to make other people's days!

So, your task between now and your second *5:2* day is in two steps:

1 **Look for the dime…** pay special attention to little surprises or boosts in your routine. Notice when nice things happen, and jot them down in your Good Things Diary or notebook.

2 **Create some surprises for other people.** The simplest thing can make a difference – helping with shopping or a pushchair, passing on the free gift from the cover of your magazine to a fellow commuter, buying a coffee for the person behind you in the queue (though don't be surprised if this one makes them wary till you explain you're in a good mood).

Note down what happened in your 5:2 notes, and how it made you feel!

SIMPLIFY DAY 2

Which of the following statements makes most sense to you?

Money... makes the world go round
    or
Money... is the root of all evil
    or
The **lack of money** *is the root of all evil*
    or
A large income *is the best recipe for happiness I ever heard of.*

Where do you stand on money?

Your attitude to money will probably depend on many factors:

- Your upbringing/your parents' attitude to money.
- How much money you have right now.
- Past experiences including wealth or poverty.
- Any debts you have, or assets you own.
- The place where you live.
- The people you live with, live near and work/socialise with.

If you're struggling to pay the bills or worried about debt, then money will be a huge source of stress and unhappiness.

And even if you're not in the midst of financial difficulties, it's easy to feel fearful about your future. In many cultures, discussing money is taboo – yet we're constantly bombarded by ads to get us to spend, spend, spend!

It's tempting to imagine that we'd be happy if only we…

- earned £10,000 or $20,000 or €30,000 more per year than we do right now
- had been born into a wealthy family, or inherited a huge bequest from a distant relative
- had made better decisions in the past.

Yet, if you tried out the 'element of surprise' bonus activity at the end of the first Simplify day, you'll have confirmed that small things can make us feel richer in other ways.

Today's activities are about trying to remove as much of the emotional power from money as possible – instead we focus on making the best of what we have. It makes total sense to want financial security, but we need to stop seeing money as an end in itself, and see it instead as simply an enabler. Then we can take control of our finances, rather than letting them control us.

Who is in charge?

If you look at the people around you – or look back at periods when you've been poorer or wealthier – you'll see that it's rarely money alone that makes us happier or more miserable.

To be clear – I am not talking about the corrosive, terrifying effect that serious financial problems can have. These need to be tackled, with help from debt specialists (see Part 4: Tools for your 5:2 life on page 356 for organisations that specialise in this area).

But fears and insecurities about money can have a disproportionate effect on our well-being. I know this from personal experience. I worry a lot about debt – as a child, I remember being very aware of financial issues in the family, and as a result I have an ingrained terror of bankruptcy. Ever since I've had control of my own finances I've been extremely cautious.

In contrast, my partner is very generous with money and gets quite irritated by my caution… On the plus side, in the time we've been together, I think our ways have rubbed off on each other. He's now likely to look for bargains – and I am more likely to splash out a bit on treats for myself and others now and then.

I'm no saint – but by becoming aware of my natural financial tendencies, I've been able to make better decisions and change my attitude.

5:2 MYTH-BUSTING

DOES MONEY BUY YOU HAPPINESS OR NOT?

Charles Dickens sums it up best for me. In his novel, *David Copperfield*, published in 1849, he wrote:

Annual income twenty pounds, annual expenditure nineteen six, **result happiness.**

Annual income twenty pounds, annual expenditure twenty pound ought and six, **result misery.**

The coinage might have changed, but the message hasn't: *debt makes you unhappy*. But how much spare cash do you need to earn or have to produce the opposite effect?

One famous US study estimated that **increases in income do make us happy, but only up to a threshold** of around $75,000 (around €55,500 or £46,000) – after that, it has no more effect. Other studies suggest that even though wealth has grown in the US since 1950, people don't rate themselves as any happier.

Another influential piece of American research found that **it's *relative* earnings that matter** – if your neighbour earns £25,000 and you earn £35,000, chances are you will be happier than him or her.

And yet another study, this time from Australia, suggests that while money might not make us happier, **people who *are* happier are likely to be more productive and earn more.** Is it chicken or egg? Your guess is as good as mine.

That's why the Dickens quote seems most useful. But there's another piece of work I find telling: the finding from a study by the London School of Economics which suggests that **when we fixate on money, then that fixation gives it the power to make us happy or unhappy**. When we focus on other things that are sources of well-being – especially family and friends, as we explored in the Connect chapter – then our income or savings (or lack of them) have far less impact.

So, for our first activity, we're going to look not at how much money we have right now, but what wealth – or freedom from worry about money – would mean to you. Then our challenge will help you gain control of your spending, your saving, or both.

Key Activity, Simplify Day 2
if I were a rich man (or woman)…

This activity will pinpoint what's at the heart of your dreams or worries around money – and help you begin to identify ways you can enjoy the things you really want without having to blow the budget.

Step 1

Let's pretend you've won the lottery. At the time of writing, this week's EuroMillions lottery jackpot is £12 million (that's around $19.4m or €14.3m). So, for a moment, let's imagine – *it's you!*

Set your phone/timer for 5 minutes and write down what you'd do with the money! Don't think too much about how it all joins up – just write down ideas and draw images that pop into your mind. Some of it might repeat stuff you dreamed of in the first week but that doesn't matter.

You probably won't need much help imagining this, but just in case…

- What would you buy? A flat in central London or a beach house in Bali? A classic Rolls Royce or a Tiffany tiara?
- Where would you go? Tour the world on a cruise ship? Take a gang of friends to New Zealand? Fly to the Moon?
- Where would you live? Who with?
- What would you do to make your own life or others' lives easier or better? Pay for medical treatment? Hire a butler? Buy a dog?
- Would you give up work, or would you miss your colleagues?

- What would you do with the rest of your life? Take it easy? Set up a charity? Climb a mountain on every continent?

Step 2

Dreaming is fun, but Step 2 is where the real work begins in order to work out what money means to you, deep down. We're using the questions:

- Why?
- What would that give you?

Pick the answers from above that excite you the most and for each one, ask why you said that – and what that dream would give you. Here's an example:

- **I want to buy a flat in central London.**
  Why? What would that give you?
- **A base nearer to where the life is.**
  Why? What would that give you?
- **Less time travelling to work and the places I like.**
  Why? What would that give you?
- **I'd be able to go to the theatre or clubs without worrying about the last train. Plus, less travelling would mean more time with family doing what I want to do instead of arriving home tired and late.**

Straight away, you've identified some of the aspects of your life that are about more than money. Yes, if you won the lottery, then getting a train home probably wouldn't be an issue but we're aiming to get at the truth or the benefits *behind* what money can buy – in this case, more nights out and more time.

Do this for each of the answers that felt most exciting, and keep asking those two questions – *Why? What would that give you?* – until you feel you've got to the heart of your response.

Step 3

Look at your answers. What do they tell you about what money means – look beyond the objects and see what they tell you about what would make you happy.

Can you find a way to make these happen without winning the lottery – by making other changes, or spending less money?

So in this example you might consider:

- Going to matinees or local theatre groups where the last train doesn't matter
- Arranging to treat a friend to a great night out in town in return for sleeping on their sofa
- Longer-term, seeing if you could make lifestyle changes, like looking for work closer to home, so you have more time and energy for your family.

Key Activity
feedback

That last activity is *not* a magic wand. And if you are concerned about serious debt, or losing your job, maybe it seems an irrelevance.

But we so often postpone happiness and changes until we have more money or have sorted certain things out in our lives: yet perhaps *we'll* never be rich, and what a waste to put things off until then. The activity is designed to show that the key is identifying what's *behind* the items you covet or the millionaire lifestyle that looks so perfect.

Remember: money is simply a tool

Money is not good or evil. It can't be moral or immoral (OK, a few people do believe that money shouldn't exist at all but I want to stay practical here).

The money we exchange daily doesn't have any 'true' value (unless you have a pirate chest full of gold doubloons). The coins and notes are simply tokens we exchange for goods and services – a wallet full of IOUs from the bank.

Money is there to enable us to do the things we want to do – yet so many of us choose to bury our heads in the sand and never quite know how much we have, or how much we owe. It may be uncomfortable to see the figures in black and white, but it's time to seize the day and face the truth. Time for one of our most challenging challenges yet!

Challenge, Simplify Day 2
take control of your money

The basic principle, whether you're in the red or in the black, is that you should pay as little interest as possible on your loans, and gain as much interest as possible on your savings.

At the time of writing, interest rates are very low in most countries, so it's even more important to be aware of what you owe, what you save and what you spend. There's no point having money in a savings account paying 1% interest if you're paying 18% on old credit card debts or a truly scary percentage on payday loans. But it's not always simple – if you take money out of an account without giving notice, you might lose all the interest you've earned.

The following are merely general guidelines so please do your own investigations before making a decision about your finances! I'm not an financial adviser or professional, just another consumer making sense of the money maze.

The options are all based on making better use of your cash by:

- spending less/getting better value or
- saving more or
- realising assets.

And they follow those basic principles: assess your position, minimise your interest charges, maximise your income from interest and other sources and make your money count:

A **Be a bean-counter:** assess your finances.

B **Be a loan-buster:** borrow at the best rate, plan to clear debts.

C **Be a savings-switcher:** maximise your interest.

D **Be a penny-pincher:** spend more wisely.

E **Be a free-loader:** find ways to get something for nothing.

F **Be an e-trader/e-guru:** share your skills or offload your clutter, for money.

G **Be a good giver/lovely lender:** help your spare cash make a difference.

If you're really fearful about your overall financial health, start with Be a bean-counter and be aware that **no single half-hour challenge can make up for months or even years of ignoring your financial situation**. The point, as with so much in this book, is to **make a start**.

If you feel overwhelmed, reread the details of the Pomodoro Technique I outlined in Week 1 on page 53 – financial admin is boring and can be daunting if you're allergic to figures, but it has one advantage over other major tasks like job change: regaining control of your money naturally breaks down into smaller tasks as you work your way through the list.

Of course, if you're a paragon of financial virtue already, you can skip Be a bean-counter and go to the most relevant option for you.

Option A Be a bean-counter

This could be the biggest challenge in this book, if you've never taken control of your money. But the results could also be life-changing.

Your aim is to discover:

- What you own.
- What you owe.
- How much you currently spend on everyday essentials.
- How much you currently spend on luxuries (or what financial types call 'discretionary purchases').

Find a large table – or use the floor – and lay out all your financial information into separate piles, including:

- statements: current account statements, credit card statements, loan statements, savings and pension statements;
- bills: regular bills like electricity, water, gas, council tax/local taxes, insurances;
- receipts: for food shopping, petrol/gasoline, events, entertainment.

Use a spreadsheet of your own, ordinary pen and paper with coloured highlighters – or try a download like these at moneysavingexpert.com.

If you can't leave the piles where they are in between sessions – or don't want others to see them – then plastic wallets or a ring-binder with different sections will help you keep organised – and I find simply having a ring binder marked 'Finances' already makes you feel more in control!

It may be that your finances are so complex – and difficult to face – that you need help, and there is plenty available – see Part 4: Tools for your 5:2 life on page 356 for more information.

Once you have the overview, you can work your way through all or any of the next options.

Option B Be a loan-buster

Shakespeare wrote 'neither a borrower nor a lender be'. – but, for once, his wisdom doesn't really transfer to the modern day, because the cost of living in the 21st century means loans are unavoidable for most of us, whether you need a mortgage, credit card or car loan.

Even when interest rates are at record lows, borrowing money is expensive – so cutting your borrowing, or finding a cheaper way to do it, can make financial sense.

Online comparison sites or best-buy tables in newspapers are the best source of up-to-date information… and in many cases switching to cheaper loans or mortgages can be relatively simple and save you plenty.

1 **Look at all your borrowing** – mortgage, credit card
   and any loans including short-term/payday loans – and
   search the small-print for the APR – annual percentage
   rate. Short-term loans are usually the scariest and debts
   escalate quickly if not paid off. Don't forget overdrafts too
   – unauthorised ones often have punishing rates.

2   **Prioritise the loans with the highest APR** *and* those
    where you are behind on repayments and are incurring
    penalties. If you are in arrears, *call the company* instead of
    hoping they'll forget about you. They won't, and the debt
    will keep increasing. Ask if the lender can switch you to a
    better product while you pay it off.

3   Finding **a lower-rate credit card deal** and transferring
    your balance is an option if you are not overdue on loans
    or credit cards. Use online calculators to see whether
    shifting large credit card debts onto a low APR deal will
    be worth the switching fee that's usually charged.

4   **Mortgages are usually the largest loans we have** – and
    so there's the potential to save a lot of money over the
    length of the loan by getting a better deal or making
    overpayments. You do need to take into account any fees
    your existing lender might charge if you switch – and the
    legal costs of transferring: try using an online calculator to
    work out costs. In some cases, if you have savings that aren't
    earning interest – or you are self-employed and need to put
    money aside for the taxman – then an offset mortgage can
    be useful. You 'offset' your savings against the loan so you
    only pay mortgage interest on the outstanding amount,
    but you can access your savings if you need to. You gain
    because the money you're not paying in mortgage interest is
    greater than what you'd earn in a savings account.

Option C Be a saving-switcher

Switch the focus now to your savings or investments.

1   **Look for the rates** on all your accounts – including
    current/checking accounts, savings accounts, regular

savings accounts, government accounts/ISAs and Premium Bonds.

2 **Prioritise the largest amounts** – they need to be working hardest for you and you may be able to get a better rate if you consolidate your savings. But bear in mind that different countries and banks vary in the protection offered if your bank gets fails, so try not to exceed that.

3 **Stay current!** You don't have to stick with the same bank you've saved with since you were a kid. It's easy to find banks with the best customer service – check ratings online – and many will even pay you to switch. Plus it can all be done electronically which saves most of the hassle.

4 **Review old accounts** – if you were tempted by an introductory offer, make sure it hasn't expired and that you aren't now on an uncompetitive rate. It's a good idea to repeat this exercise once a year, especially as financial institutions can take advantage of customer laziness.

5 **Check the small-print before withdrawing any money** – notice accounts may penalise you if you don't give enough notice, and UK ISAs can be transferred, but only by using a specific route, otherwise you lose tax-free status.

Option D Be a penny-pincher

Thriftiness has become cool... so long as you don't become obsessed (remember my cautionary tale about time wasted comparing car breakdown schemes on page 49).

Your two main targets for penny-pinching savings should be large, one-off payments – and regular bills.

1 **One-off payments** like insurances can vary hugely for the same cover, and loyalty as a customer rarely pays. Make

sure too that you don't end up paying extra for monthly instalments if you can afford to pay up front. Think about whether you really need the insurance. Insuring a toaster that you can afford to replace is a waste of money – but not insuring your home or car is very high-risk. Also check your bank accounts for insurances you've forgotten you had, they could be for things you don't even own anymore.

2   Next, think about your **shopping bills and regular expenses** – ideally gather receipts for food shops and daily lunches/coffees and look at the things you buy most often. If you want to cut down, you could:

   a   Try one of the budget supermarkets (Aldi in the UK recently won Best Supermarket awarded by the Consumers' Association) – the products are often high-quality, though the shops are no-frills.

   B   Whichever supermarket you go to, consider own brands – try them out if they represent a big saving. (If you have fussy foodies in the house, decant products into the branded containers and see if they notice the difference.)

   C   For daily expenses like coffees or sandwiches, do some sums or use the Demotivator from the Money Saving Expert site (moneysavingexpert.com/shopping/demotivator) to show how much cutting out one sandwich, buying a smaller coffee, or – for the ultimate saving – bringing your own, could save you over a year.

   D   Join the local library – free books! Free events! Free culture! What's not to love? And it'll help you connect with your local community.

E   Try out our Bonus Activity – the 5:2 spending diet
on page 143!

Thriftiness is all the rage on the net, too, so check out great blogs like athriftymrs.com and somehowwemanage.com for more inspiration.

Option E Be a free-loader

Free-loading can be fun – and many companies encourage you to try their stuff for free, especially if you're a prolific social networker because your recommendation can create a buzz that money can't buy. Here are a few fast ideas to sign up for (but do be prepared for lots of annoying emails once companies have your email address!):

1   **Cashback sites:** this is the easiest way to make a little extra from purchases you'd make anyway, simply by clicking through from a site like Topcashback.co.uk or Quidco.com in the UK, and StartHere.com.au in Australia. The best cashback tends to come on big purchases or commitments like mobile phone contracts or insurances and you shouldn't make choices based on cashback, but it can be a nice addition. You could make £200+ in a year's purchases for the family.

2   **Cinema previews:** movie distributors often arrange free previews to build excitement around a new release, though these are most often in the bigger cities and tend to be in the morning at weekends, or early evening during the week. You join the mailing list and then have to respond very fast!

3   **Product trials:** you can sign up for 'buzz' campaigns run by consumer research agencies who will send you anything from cosmetics to washing powders to gadgets to try out, either for free or reduced price. They rely on you then using 'word of mouth' to talk about the products. Or you might get invited onto a focus group to give your views. The forums on the Moneysavingexpert website are a good place to start to find reputable companies.

4   **Mystery shopping:** yes, you can get a free lunch... so long as you don't mind snooping on the restaurant and reporting back. I've done this – I've even written three novels about it, including *The Secret Shopper's Revenge*. It can be hassly in terms of paperwork, but it's fun and you can actually feel that you're raising customer service standards, and rewarding good service when you find it. You can also earn a small fee for many assignments. Again, check forums to find out which companies offer good assignments – and never pay up front to an agency.

5   **DIY free-loading:** it's not all about big corporations. Try out DIY free-loading by organising thrifty social events, from a clothes swap with all your friends, to a cocktail night where you all bring a bottle of something you brought back from a holiday duty-free shop and have no idea how to use!

Option F Be an e-trader/e-guru
Selling your stuff – or your skills – has never been easier.

- eBay is the obvious way to do it, but if you have a specialist skill or unusual objects, then you may get better prices for your products or heirlooms on other sites like crafster.org for home-made items.

- Can you teach or pass on a skill, whether it's crochet, book-keeping or conversational Spanish? The chances to earn money from offering online tutoring, or bidding to provide services, have been opened up by sites like skillshare.com/classes and peopleperhour.com.

Option G Be a good giver/a lovely lender

If you have money to spare, then charities will always want to receive donations. But you don't necessarily have to *give* the money away – you can also invest your money in a way that encourages businesses or helps people find their financial feet. Please note I haven't checked out the detail of all these sites, so do your research before parting with any money!

- Angel investment sites: you can invest through sites like angelinvestmentnetwork.co.uk or for more creative projects, kickstarter.com which also offers overseas projects which can aid development
- The idea of fundingcircle.com is to pool your money to loan to small businesses in the UK.
- Or think local, by investing in credit unions, which offer ethical savings based in your local community: findyourcreditunion.co.uk

Finally… don't worry, be 'appy

The range of apps and websites to help with your finances is vast, and growing all the time. There are privacy and security issues, of course, but the apps that help you change your behaviour in small ways – much as we work on making small changes two days a week – can be fun and motivating without being off-putting.

Obviously these apps do change, but at the time of writing, I like:

- Mint – available online, for Android and IoS: mint.com – is a very thorough financial planning and monitoring tool, which can help you budget and save for something specific.
- Manilla – available online, for Android and IoS: manilla. com – has similar tools but is best for helping you to keep track of bills and payments leaving your account.

Challenge: feedback

If you're at the 'bean counting' stage and have taken your first step towards being in control of your money, then congratulations!

Whatever stage you're at in your financial life, this bonus activity encourages you to be mindful about your spending. It's one you can try any time you like.

Bonus Activity, Simplify Day 2
the 5:2 spending diet

The 5:2 Diet itself involves eating just 25% of your daily calorie allowance for a couple of days a week – to cut your overall energy consumption *and* make you aware of what you're eating the rest of the time.

So, for this activity, we're cutting down on daily *spending* to reduce financial consumption on the day *and* make you more aware of your spending the rest of the time. It's simple:

- Work out what you spend most days – and cut your budget to 25% of that (or if you're really keen, down to nothing), for one or two days in the coming week.
- Plan how you're going to achieve this, look at the 'Be a penny-pincher' option on page 138. You can either see this as a way to save for the future – a money diet! – or an experiment to see whether you enjoy existing on less!
- Jot down some notes on how you find it – writing down what you spend can be a great way of raising awareness of what you really want versus what you buy without thinking…
- Most exitingly, decide what you'd like to do with the money you save – whether it's something beautiful, useful or exciting, you've earned it.

Simplify Week: key points

Here's a summary of our key points from this week:

- Simplify your life by clearing mental and physical clutter to help you see your goals more clearly.
- Making small changes to your physical environment can support changes to your routine.
- Delegating tasks you hate is easier than you think – and can buy you extra time.
- Money is simply a tool – and only by taking control and being aware of it can you keep it in its place!
- Being clear about what's more important to you in your life can help you deal with any shortages or excesses of money.

Week 4

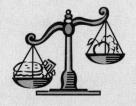

The way to get started is to quit talking and begin doing.

Walt Disney

Week 4: checking in

Is your life suitably simplified after last week's activities and challenges? Here's a quick checklist to help you review your progress.

- Are you enjoying the space you cleared with the 'five senses' approach? It's easy to expand out from that initial room when you feel in the mood.

- Have you tried the 5:2 spending diet? If it helps motivate you, why not work out something you'd like to save for on those 5:2 days?

- My tip: if you're decluttering and are in two minds about different items or pieces of clothing, put them in a bag or box in the attic or under the stairs. Mark a date in your diary – perhaps six months to a year ahead – to check the box. If you haven't needed or missed the items, take the bag straight to the charity shop or recycling centre!

Move

THIS WEEK'S AIM:
To start moving – physically and mentally – so you have more energy, confidence & drive to get where you want to be

Introduction

We're moving forward this week – as we think about health, energy levels and fitness. If the idea of exercise makes you groan, I promise there's nothing dull about this week's activities and challenges.

On Move Day 1, we'll focus on finding out what you enjoy doing – and get moving. And on Move Day 2, we'll explore ways to get more active in your daily routine, without even really noticing…

MOVE QUIZ

As with previous weeks, this quiz isn't *exactly* scientific, but it's a great warm-up to kick-start our new theme…

This week: **how you move**

1 Zoom back in time to PE lessons at school. Were you?
   A   The last kid to be picked for the team.
   B   The kid doing the picking – always team captain!
   C   Somewhere in the middle.
   D   Still lurking in the changing room, trying to forge your mum's signature on the sick note.

2 What is your job and lifestyle like?
   A   Sedentary – I'd like to do more, but I've never found an activity I enjoy.
   B   Very active – I like to be fit and to push myself.
   C   I enjoy being on the move but how much exercise I get depends on what else is going on in my life. It can't be top priority.
   D   I'm a couch potato – I don't believe in wasting energy!

3 How does your body make you feel?
   A   Concerned – I want to be fitter for the sake of my health.
   B   Happy – I love how it feels to move around and try new sports.
   C   OK – it does the job well and I only creak or ache occasionally.
   D   It's not something I think about… unless my doctor forces me to.

If you found yourself drawn to…

Mostly As: you're talking my language. You're definitely not a natural athlete but you want to feel fitter. Don't worry – I've been like this and found lots of new ways to make moving around more fun.

Mostly Bs: Top marks! You're good at this fitness business. But there's still plenty in this chapter to inspire you to even greater things.

Mostly Cs: your heart's in the right place, but your trainers are at the back of the wardrobe. However, you don't need trainers, or a gym membership, to make a difference to your health and energy levels. Read on!

Mostly Ds: time to get moving. You need some motivation – and the facts in this chapter should be enough to persuade you that you can change your habits, with very little effort.

MOVE DAY 1

Exercise is one of the words I hate most in the English language.

To me, exercise suggests something dull and relentless and potentially painful. I'm picturing Lycra-clad humiliations, Jane Fonda in a leotard demanding that I *feel the burn, a*nd the smell of sweaty socks and damp gym kit left too long in the bottom of a rucksack.

No wonder the idea of 'exercising' for half an hour five times a week *for the rest of our lives* (which is the minimum recommended by the NHS and others) can be a tough one for many of us to take on board.

But if I swap the word exercising for the word 'moving', things start to look rather different.

Moving is about progress, about taking a step forward, having a purpose. About changing things, or dancing like no one's watching, or going places.

You can move anywhere, any time. There's no special equipment required, no one shouting at you, no guilt.

Human beings are designed to move...

Look at any group of young children. Moving around is an instinct, and they'll do it any way they can, starting by grabbing for things that are out of reach, then shimmying, pushing, pulling and using every means they can to get to new places and explore the world around them.

Most have naturally good posture, with flexible limbs and the ability to twist and change direction faster than us! They're full of energy – though when they sleep, they *really* sleep, to recharge their batteries for the next bout of racing around!

Wouldn't you love to get back the excitement and energy you had as a young child, always reaching for the next thing?

Rethinking how you move is the answer.

With that in mind, today we're going to mix things up a bit – and start with our challenge, instead of our key activity.

Because I want you to get moving!

Challenge, Move Day 1: go!

Either right now or by the end of today, I want you to commit to moving more than usual! I'm not talking a sprint, or a full-on aerobics session, but simply something that you'll enjoy and that gets the blood flowing. Aim for 20–25 minutes of activity, or more if you can… (and more good news: you don't *have* to do it all in one go!)

IMPORTANT HEALTH WARNING

If you have any concerns or health issues, please do see your doctor before doing anything that counts as exercise or includes movements or activities you don't normally do. I want you to feel better, not worse!

Ready? Here's what you can do today:

- **Love the outdoors?** Borrow your neighbour's dog and give it a run round the local park.
- **Make your commute more energising:** Get off at least one bus/train/tube stop earlier than usual on your journey home, and time yourself. Next time, walk faster. (Top tip: if you can manage to get off before the next fare zone, you'll save money too.)
- **Involve your family or friends:** Pick the kids up from school on foot instead of in the car (it'll get them in the habit of moving too) or arrange to meet a friend for a walk instead of automatically choosing to go to the café.
- **Kill two birds with one stone:** Do some vigorous gardening – digging, mowing, hauling rubbish to the recycling (great if you like to achieve something while getting fitter). Or clean the house as fast as humanly possible, without tripping over the vacuum cleaner lead – get out of breath!
- **Lift your mood while you work out:** Put on your most upbeat music on the MP3 player and walk/jog to the nearest green space or dance frantically around your living room.

How hard should I work?

The guideline for adults in good health already is to work hard enough so you're slightly out of breath for the duration of your session, but still able to hold a conversation.

Another way to gauge how hard you are working is with the Perceived Rate of Exertion (or PRE – this is a simplified version of the Borg scale which is used to estimate how hard the heart is working in a medical setting). Simply estimate how hard you're working on a scale of 1 to 10 where 1 is sitting down and 10 is the hardest you can possibly work, without collapsing!

Ideally, you should be aiming for around 5 or 6 when you start a new regime. What most people find is that your PRE adapts rapidly as your fitness improves – in other words, very soon you'll be able to do more vigorous activities, for a lower PRE score. Which is super-encouraging…

All ready to get moving? Or maybe you need a little extra motivation?

Dreaded consequences as a motivational tool

Most of us respond more to the carrot than the stick: that is, we prefer to gain rewards than avoid punishment. But if you're resisting any positive change, consider the stick…

- If you don't do the activity you've committed to doing, you have to choose a penalty that you hate even more.
- The most motivating penalties are often financial. So, list the charities or causes that you *really* dislike. Political parties are good for this – find ones that take the opposite view of something you feel very strongly about…
- Make a pledge that if you don't complete the activity, you'll donate a sum of money to that cause. Ouch!

But the penalty doesn't have to be financial – it could be:
- cleaning the oven
- removing the rust from the barbecue
- offering to clear the cat poo out of your neighbour's garden

- cooking a food you really hate but your partner/kids love, ideally something very smelly!

What matters is that it has to be something you'd hate more than doing the activity.

Does going for that lovely walk now sound a bit less of a chore? If you can, go and complete your challenge right now.

Challenge: feedback

After your challenge, jot down a few notes about how it made you feel – before, during and after. Rate your mood out of 10 before, during and after. This will help you plan other activities – and see progress.

As an example, here's how I felt.

Before the gym:

- Physical: sluggish. Cold feet and hands. Quite hunched from writing to deadline. 6/10
- Mental: I don't have the energy to go to the gym. When I get there I'll struggle to run, it was hard last time. I have too much to do. I never seem to achieve as much as I need to. 6/10

After the gym:

- Physical effects: My circulation has improved, blood's pumping – and I also like it when I stop and notice how quickly my body recovers! 9/10
- Mental: Wahey! I feel great to have done something physical

154

when my job is sedentary; I managed to push myself further than I expected and keep going when at first I didn't think I'd be able to. I definitely feel very happy and pleased I've managed to get out there and do it. Now I'm ready to tackle the other stuff I've been avoiding! 10/10

How does that compare with how *you* felt before and after? If you're new to regular activity, you may find it's harder to get motivated to start with. But that changes quite quickly: I no longer need to convince myself to go to the gym because I know how good I'll feel afterwards!

5:2 MYTH-BUSTING

THE TRUTH ABOUT MOOD, EXERCISE AND THE RUNNER'S HIGH?

Are endorphins all they're cracked up to be?

Why does exercise make us feel good? You might have heard the phrase, 'runner's high' to describe the state of euphoria that follows any prolonged exercise, not just running. For a long time, we've assumed this is caused by the release of endorphins, the body's own equivalent of morphine.

More recently, some researchers have developed a different theory, believing it's the brain's *cannabinoid* system at work, which, you guessed it, can produce cannabis-like effects on our bodies. The research continues but the precise biology doesn't matter to me – what does matter is that exercise can truly give us a natural high!

What about exercise as an anti-depressant?

We know anecdotally that many people report feeling great after exercise. But does that mean people with depressive illness or other mental health issues will be helped by moving more?

Before I started looking at the research on this, I expected there to be much stronger evidence for the anti-depressant effects of exercise. The confusing issue is that it's hard to separate cause from effect. Does exercise help to *prevent* depression, or is it that people who are clinically depressed therefore *lack* the motivation and energy to get moving?

Exercise may certainly boost resilience to stress and anxiety, and a 'prescription' of exercise for people suffering from depression has shown good results (see the Resources section from page 352 for a link a more detailed analysis).

There are many exciting research projects going on to tease out the relationship between mood and exercise, sleep, genes, brain chemistry and even the potential benefits of intermittent fasting like the 5:2 Diet. In the meantime, we can say without doubt that moving more will:

- increase our sense of achievement and feeling of control
- give us a break from niggling worries by making us focus on what our bodies are doing
- increase social contact if we enjoy team games, or literally widen our horizons if we exercise outdoors.

Getting personal: why finding the right activity is the key to success

As our quiz at the start of this week shows, we all come to movement with different memories, abilities and motivations. Tapping into the things we enjoy is, I believe, the most vital part of making movement part of your life. Choose the right activity, and you're more likely to make the effort to fit it in. Choose the wrong one, and the odds against continuing are *very* high.

You might have noticed that in the challenge, I listed the extra benefits that you can gain from the different suggested activites – like boosting your mood, or involving family and friends. Right now, we're going to explore in more detail how *you* can find activities that suit your lifestyle and your mood, as well as your body.

Key Activity, Move Day 1
my movement DNA

Step 1: 15 minutes
Think about the kinds of activity you enjoy – and the kind you'd run a mile from. I want you to work out where you are on each of these lines below and then jot down some notes about your reaction to each question. (You can download this at www.the5-2dietbook.com/freebies)

I--------------------------------------I--------------------------------------I
I love the great outdoors,   Brrrr – can't stand the
whatever the weather   cold or the wet

I--------------------------------------I--------------------------------------I
Team games are fun –   Team games are hell –
I love working together   I hate the peer pressure

I--------------------------------------I--------------------------------------I
I love to compete   I prefer to compete against
against others   my own personal bests

I--------------------------------------I--------------------------------------I
I feel great when I can measure or count   I prefer to focus on how I feel
my achievement in time or information   and my mood after an experience

I--------------------------------------I--------------------------------------I
I already move a lot in   I am pretty inactive or
my spare or leisure time   unfit at the moment

I--------------------------------------I--------------------------------------I
I can afford to invest a little   I don't have a budget/I don't
money in being active   want to spend anything

I--------------------------------------I--------------------------------------I
I love moving for its own sake   I'd prefer to achieve something
                                                                               else at the same time

I--------------------------------------I--------------------------------------I
I don't have any current health   I do need medical advice or support
issues that would restrict me   before starting a new routine

Finished? Now jot down any activities you remember enjoying when you were younger – either as a child or a younger adult. Whether it's synchronised swimming or playground skipping, get it down.

Finally, take a look at your notes – what do they suggest to you in terms of activities you might enjoy? We have lots of suggestions coming right up...

Step 2: 10 minutes

Are some trends emerging? Some may seem obvious: it's a bad idea to force yourself to take up netball if you hate team games, and a great idea to start walking in the countryside if you love getting muddy!

But other subtler factors are at play here, too – some activities will really appeal if you want to see numbers that will improve rapidly as you get fitter, whereas other people are motivated more by the buzz they feel from working out or getting back to nature. And then there's the practical side: the time of year, your budget (or lack of it) and any existing injuries or health issues that might restrict your choice of activity. Though that needn't stand in your way.

Taking your own preferences into account, I want you to plan your next Move activity, for the second of this week's 5:2 days.

- Aim for 25 minutes' activity in total.
- Look at the ideas below (or on page 152), choose one of these or one of your own.
- Write it in your diary and note it on your 5:2 planner, if you're using it.
- Make it an appointment you can't afford to miss (and commit to a dreaded consequence if you do).

More Move ideas:

- Go to the DVD drawer and **find that fitness video** you bought two years ago but is still in its wrapper… or go online to a site like sparkpeople.com or youtube.com where you can search for and watch workouts on your tablet or laptop. Preview a couple of the routines so you're ready to go – some presenters are so irritating that you might end up preferring a dreaded consequence!

- Is there a local gym near you? Many offer **free one day passes** so call or go online to sign up for one right now. If you can, give yourself time to enjoy the facilities – often they'll include a pool, sauna or steam room to help you relax (plus saunas may raise the metabolism by up to 20% as you use energy maintaining the correct temperature!).

- **Invest in a pedometer** – on Day 2 I will share the story of how I fell in love with mine!

- Download the **Couch to 5K podcasts** from the NHS or other providers – these take you on a structured, safe training programme, even if you can't run without getting out of breath. In just two months you go from 30 second bursts to running for half an hour at a time…

- Keep an eye out on what's available in your area – if you're looking for ways to increase your movement, you might be surprised at the possibilities you spot. It's another example of the Puppy Effect (see page 58) in action.

Key Activity

feedback

Done? Diarised?

On Move Day 2, we'll explore ways to increase your chances of sticking to good habits, but scheduling an appointment is the first step.

Now that's all organised, settle back and prepare to feel smug about what you've achieved today... and enjoy a relaxing and creative end to your session.

Bonus (Optional) Activity, Move Day 1

move mood board

This activity can grow, week by week – and it's perfect if you need a bit of recovery time after being active! As a writer, I don't know if I agree that a picture really does paint a thousand words, but great images can certainly inspire us all.

So, you're going to start a mood board.

- You can use either an online service/app like Pinterest – which has a great community element, too – or a large piece of card, scissors, glue and a stack of magazines. Evernote is another app that can work across your computer/Mac, phone and tablet.

If online:

- Look for images of the activities, locations and feelings you hope for with a new, more active life.
- Add your own images, uploaded from your computer, as you try out new things, or find other activities in the local area.
- Expand the board – or create a new one – adding how you want to feel and look – clothes, locations, equipment that might help you be more active.
- Once you have your account set up, you can display images across all your devices if you want to be inspired wherever you are.

If you choose to make a physical mood board/collage:

- Go through a stack of magazines and look for a few key images – but then keep your eye out wherever you are for more print images, including postcards, flyers for classes, labels from your new trainers – anything visual that helps you record your journey.
- If you have children, involve them in the process too – ask them to draw pictures of the activities you're trying, or the 'new you' (of course, you could scan and upload these to a Pinterest board if you want).
- Keep the board somewhere to inspire you – inside the wardrobe, on the fridge door.

Don't stop with one board – once you're in the swing of it, you could develop one for each of the sections in *5:2 Your Life,* as a visual diary, to record what you've done.

Cool down...

That's it for today – have you scheduled some movement or activity for your next 5:2 day? In that case, it's time for a well-deserved rest . . .

MOVE DAY 2
mood, motivation and mini-moves

How are you feeling? Raring to get moving? Today we're talking micro-movements, good habits and why standing up is the new sitting down!

But, for now, let's start as we mean to go on – like on Day 1, we're starting with the challenge!

Challenge, Move Day 2
move!

Step 1

Last time, you came up with a movement-based activity for today, so hopefully you've got something fun lined up.

So all you need to do now is go and do it!

If you didn't plan something, not to worry. You can simply:

- repeat what you did on the first Move day
- get onto YouTube.com, fitnesstv.co.uk or sparkpeople.com and find an online workout

Or… remember, you could always carry out something that counts as a dreaded consequence (see page 153)? No? Thought that wouldn't appeal!

Step 2

When you're back, write down how you felt. Remember to score your mood out of 10: before, during and after. Have a think about what might be *behind* how you're feeling. Being aware of your motivations will help you turn moving more into the very best kind of habit!

The many, many pluses of moving more

Movement, or exercise, is about much more than toned pecs. It's about physical and mental well-being, good health and staying active for as long as we possibly can.

- It's great for your heart – and aerobic exercise (the kind that leaves you a little short of breath) can reduce high blood pressure, if you do it often enough. It can also reduce the risk of suffering a stroke and reduce the symptoms of Type 2 diabetes.
- It's great for your bones – women in particular are at risk from osteoporosis (a reduction in bone density and therefore strength) but weight-bearing exercises like jogging or brisk walking will help reduce the risks.
- It can help manage chronic conditions including rheumatoid and osteoarthritis, and asthma.
- It can have positive effects on memory and, as we saw earlier, can reduce stress.
- It makes you feel great!

WHAT EXERCISE CAN'T DO...

However, this next part might surprise you. It certainly shocked me!

Most of us believe that exercise will help us lose weight. Yet when we join a gym or try out a running machine, it can be astonishing to see how few calories we burn, even when we take the most intense exercise.

It depends on your weight, gender and age but a woman weighing 10 stone/63.5 kilograms will use around this number of calories per 30 minutes of each activity:

Writing	34
Ironing	71
Shopping	76
Cooking	84
Housework	92
Sex	134
Pilates (intermediate)	164
Gardening	172
Swimming (moderate)	193
Aerobics (high impact)	223
Jogging	223
Zumba	252
Fast cycling (12–14 mph)	277
Elliptical/cross-trainer	361

(source: www.healthstatus.com/calculate/cbc)

If you weigh more than 10 stone, you'll burn more calories than these examples, but not that much more... and when you think that a Mars bar is around 260 calories, and even a medium banana comes out at over 100, it's quite eye-opening.

The obesity epidemic vs the gym revolution

These figures do help explain something that has puzzled many people. Over the last fifty years, the populations of more affluent countries have put on weight – even though this time period has also seen the biggest growth in the exercise-as-leisure sector, with gyms and fitness videos and personal trainers more accessible than ever before.

The reasons are much debated and are almost certainly down to a combination of factors – including changes to diet, especially processed and sugary foods. There's also some evidence that extra exercise or activity may make us want to eat more to compensate – biology is powerful and our bodies want us to stay alive.

But our more sedentary lifestyles are also likely to be a factor. An hour of Zumba or cycling is great fun, and has benefits, but it's unlikely to compensate for rich foods and working in a desk job.

Luckily, there is plenty we can do to counteract an inactive work or home life – starting today!

Moving a little and moving a lot

Making the effort to be more active throughout your day can be as good for your health – and potentially even better – as doing more vigorous workouts. Recent research suggests that even if you exercise regularly, being sedentary most of the time means you're at increased risk of diabetes, heart disease and cancers.

STAND UP! SITTING DOWN IS BAD FOR YOU

One study by researchers at Leicester and Loughborough Universities in the UK analysed data from 800,000 people and concluded that the risks of premature death, especially from diabetes, were much higher in people who sat or lay down the most. Another university team found a connection between hours spent inactive, and the likelihood of disability over the age of 60.

Why? Reductions in muscle activity, circulation and metabolism are likely to play a part. Those who move or stand up more also appear to show positive effects in terms of their blood sugar. Even the experts aren't quite sure what's going on, but they do agree that not moving for extended periods is a bad thing (see the Resources section from page 352 for more on the fascinating science of standing up).

The good news? The answer is just footsteps away... and it's very *neat*.

Micro-movements – the NEAT way to stay healthy!

NEAT stands for Non-Exercise Activity Thermogenesis and means all the activities you do that aren't intended as 'exercise' but still consume energy (and burn calories!).

James Levine, a US Professor of Medicine at the Mayo Clinic, has published a book on his NEAT research, in which he says that while desk-bound workers take around 5–6,000 steps a day, more active people might manage 10,000 or more – and that building more activity into our whole day can improve health and help us shift weight.

Burning calories is only part of the story. The effects on the body *and* mind of spending the day locked in one position, over laptops or machinery, are not positive. Even our eyes get tired: they're designed to be focusing at different distances all the time, yet in modern life, we're often focused on text just a few inches from our faces. No wonder sometimes life goes a bit blurry.

We need to sit up and take notice. Or rather, *stand up* and take notice. Micro-movements can be as simple as:

- walking to buy your lunch
- taking the stairs instead of the lift
- having business meetings standing up or walking
- walking on the spot while watching TV
- cleaning, ironing, cooking
- standing up and having a really good stretch of all your muscles.

In short, most things that involve moving could be NEAT activities – and they could add up to 100s of extra calories burned during the day.

You might even have seen pictures of office workers on treadmills or step-machines built into their desks – perhaps a little extreme for most of us, but the idea is that we never stay still for too long. My colleague Peta works at a computer all day, yet since she started standing up at her desk (the computer mounted on a tower of books!), she's noticed weight loss and much, much greater energy all day long.

I find the research into the threats of a sedentary lifestyle very compelling, and have been working hard to increase my movement, helped by my love affair with my pedometer (the romance story is coming very shortly).

Research is one thing – how do you transform it into action? It's all about making movement a habit.

5:2 INSPIRATIONS

HABIT-FORMING FOR BEGINNERS

If you've ever read a book that promises you can give up a bad habit or *transform your life in 21 days*, you may think three weeks is a magical time period for transforming yourself. But the amount of time it takes to break a habit – or form a better one – is very personal, and depends on how central that old habit was to your life, or how rewarding the new habit might be.

Habits are automatic behaviours – things we do without really thinking, because they've become part of our routine. Think about eating at certain times of day, brushing your teeth, even the order that you put on or take off your clothes!

You can think of a new habit being made up of three stages: the cue, the action, the reward:

1 A **cue or trigger** that makes you carry out the new good habit: like setting an alarm to get up and go running, or leaving the house to pick the kids up from school later than usual, so you'll only arrive on time *if* you jog or powewalk.

2 The **habit or action itself:** the behaviour you want to change. Understanding *why* you want to change and what benefits it'll bring will help a great deal.

3 A **reward** after the habit or action... so long as it doesn't undermine the habit (a cigarette after the gym is not a great idea). The activity itself may bring rewards – being outdoors in the sun, or feeling fitter.

Habit helpers

To help a new habit bed in quickly, try:

- **Reminders** – something in your environment to stop you 'forgetting' – it could be as simple as leaving your trainers in the hall! I now put my gym kit on in the morning when I get up so I'm all set to go after working for three hours at my desk. Even putting on your sports bra under your work wear could be enough to remind you to go to the gym at lunchtime!

- **Helpers** – actions or items that make the new habit easier or more enjoyable, from new workout gear, to a great playlist on your MP3 or a friend running with you.

- **Penalties** – Remember those dreaded consequences from the first Move day (page 153)? If you need an extra shove, then having to do something you like less than this new habit can be a powerful motivator, so long as you *will* take the punishment!

If you want to read more about this, there's a brilliant post at sparringmind.com/good-habits which is relevant to the whole *5:2 Your Life* approach, but now it's time to put the theories to the test!

Key Activity, Move Day 2
get the habit

Step 1

- **Decide on the new habit you want to create:** it's up to you – schedule in longer periods of training or go for the NEAT approach of micro-movements?
  - *NEAT habit example*: Get up and move at least every hour (or half-hour) during your working day and your TV watching in the evening – start by doing this on your 5:2 days and, if you feel better for it, try to adopt the habit full time.
  - *Scheduled training example:* do sustained activity at least twice a week: name the day and time (for example, after work on Tuesdays and Thursdays) and the activity, for example, Zumba.
- Write down *why* you're doing it – and what the benefits will be. Be as specific as possible, to bring the idea to life.
  - How do you think you will feel when it's a regular part of your routine?
  - What physical benefits do you hope it'll bring?
  - What else might it lead to – for example, running in a race or being able to cut down on painkillers for chronic conditions?
- Find your cue or trigger:
  - *NEAT example*: a simple alarm on your phone, or reminder on your email calendar, can prompt you to move every hour.

- *Scheduled training example*: if it's a class, then the cue will be a time or alarm or a phone call from a friend. If you're going running or to the gym or doing a DVD, then make it something else – the theme music for a TV show you hate, or simply changing into your gear.
- Choose a reward:
  - *NEAT example*: keep a daily tally – when you've done eight mini-walks, staircases or stretches you could treat yourself to a hot drink or a phone call with a friend. When you've done 40 during the week, why not book a massage or buy a magazine?
  - *Scheduled training example*: reward yourself with something like a hot shower with aromatic shower gel, or a foot massage from a willing partner!

Step 2

Make it happen – and chart your progress!
- **Chart your progress** over the next week – mark on your 5:2 planner how successful you've been.
- If you find you're resistant to the new habits, look back at the checklist above to think of other ways to make the habit happen, a dreaded consequence perhaps?

Now, are you ready for my NEAT love story?

The power of (pedometer) love

The thing that has changed my activity levels more than anything else in the last few months is just over two inches (or five centimetres) long, made of black plastic and hangs onto my bra at all times.

It's a 'smart' pedometer (mine is a FitBit but there are several different brands), designed to count how many steps you take in a day (or, in my case, how few). At first I resisted paying almost £80 for a bit of plastic (there are much cheaper ones available) but I have to tell you it's been a far better investment than a pair of trainers.

The recommended number of steps per day is 10,000 (this figure originated in Japan during the 1960s – where the average household now has 3.1 pedometers!). You may think 10,000 doesn't sound many, until you realise it adds up to a distance of around 5 miles (8 kilometres) And let me tell you, it's not easy to do at first.

I didn't realise quite *how* sedentary I was till I got my pedometer. Some days, I was taking under 1,000 steps (mainly to and from the coffee machine). Well, clearly that wasn't good enough.

Before and after

Things have changed, ladies and gents. In the five months since I got my new best friend, I've walked over 1.3 million steps – a total of 600 miles or 960 kilometres – and now average 9,200 steps a day. Here's why I think it worked:

- You get 'badges' and emails when you reach a certain number of steps or stairs, which is fun and motivating.
- It records stairs as well as steps – and if you live in a Victorian cottage as I do, with no downstairs loo, you can quickly build those up!
- The element of competition against myself . . .
- And against others: I bought one for my sceptical boyfriend – he's absolutely not into gadgets, but loves it too and gets quite annoyed if he leaves it at home. Or if I beat him – yes,

you can compete against friends week by week, too.

There are a few downsides. The more expensive the pedometer, the more likely you are to put it in the hot wash. And though the clips are quite robust, I do know people who have lost them.

Pedometers also don't record how much of your movement was aerobic – i.e. got you properly out of breath – though there is a flower icon on mine that grows or wilts depending on how active I'm being. They don't record strength training or cycling either but overall, I can live with that, and the next generation of trackers do record different forms of movement.

The biggest lesson for me is about building in movement – NEAT activities as well as formal exercise. It takes a hell of a long walk to do 10,000 in one go. *Much* easier to build in lots of bursts of activity during the day – a walk to the post office, a trip round your workplace, or going to your favourite sandwich bar for lunch instead of the one just round the corner.

If you don't fancy splashing out on a new piece of kit, then there's another option: one that could cost less than the price of a cup of coffee.

'Appiness, 'appiness...

There's been a boom in health and fitness apps for phones or tablets – and we're told that our smartphones have capabilities that exceed the technology that put men on the moon! So, your mobile can easily become a fitness coach, monitoring station and pedometer all rolled into one.

Here are a few of my favourites:

- **Myfitnesspal** – helps me monitor weight, BMI, calories consumed and exercise. I found it invaluable when I started

5:2 though the calorie counts are supplied by users and are not always reliable. But it's great as a free app which covers so much ground.

- **Vital Signs** – (www.vitalsignscamera.com) this app measures your heart rate simply by using the tablet's camera to detect changes in skin colour. OK, the value of heart rate as an indicator of heart health isn't as good as, say, blood pressure, but the app is still fun and shows what could be in store in future via remote healthcare. Already, for example, pacemakers can report on heart rhythms via home modems, reducing time spent in hospital.

- **Fitstar** – (fitstar.com) is a personal training app that offers a free and a premium subscription that adapts to your current needs and capabilities, with workouts starting at seven minutes, all suitable to do at home.

I've got my eye on the Zombies, Run! app which combines a horror story with the Couch to 5K running programme that'll get you running in just a few weeks.

I also asked the fitness fans on the 5:2 fitness Facebook group for their recommendations:

- Amber likes ACTIVE couch to 5k: 'You can choose voice-over and it works with other apps and is user friendly. I like the Nike app – I compete against friends and measure my own goals but Runkeeper and Mapmyrun also do this well.'

- She also recommends this 'Never Give Up' video for motivation http://youtu.be/qX9FSZJu448.

- Rebecca suggests: 'Map my Fitness and Zombies Run are good, and Adidas miCoach lets you sign up to training plans and has Jonny Wilkinson's voice to spur you on!'

- Andie is one of the many, many fans of Jillian Michael's 30-

Day Shred – 'The programme is not for the faint-hearted! But free on you tube!' http://youtu.be/1Pc-NizMgg8.
- Lucy really likes RunDouble for C25k Couchto5K.

If you're inspired to try something new, but want to keep costs down, then today's Bonus Activity is for you.

Bonus Activity, Move Day 2
what can you do for a fiver?

Varying your movement regime will keep you interested, but that doesn't have to mean spending lots on personal trainers or fancy gyms. A little can go a long way when it comes to fitness.

So your bonus activity – should you choose to accept this – involves giving yourself a budget of £5 and seeing how far it can take you. Let's face it, a celeb fitness trainer wouldn't do up a single shoelace for that, but with a little *5:2 Your Life* magic, we can do wonders.

Here are some ideas:
- Download a fiver's worth of apps onto your phone or tablet to inspire and motivate you.
- Go hunting for bargain DVDs on eBay, Amazon or at a car boot sale. You can often get them for a really low cost when people have had a clear out.
- Spend it on a class you've never tried before, anything from bokwa to ballroom dancing. Look for a class at your nearest church hall or community centre – try something new that sounds fun (and you'll get also be getting all the extra

benefits of meeting people locally that I outlined in the Connect week!).

- Try out a boot camp, martial art or boxing-based class. They're not for everyone – personally it's my idea of hell – but many people find these fun and a fantastic antidote to any frustrations during the working week!
- Buy some bulbs or seedlings and use them to kick-start a garden makeover. There's nothing like a good dig to get the heart pumping. Or look for outdoor fitness and activity sessions run by conservation groups where you help improve the environment while getting fit!
- Anyone for tennis? Council tennis courts cost under £5 (and sometimes free) to hire and are sociable, too. Look for leagues near you. Most have a beginners' group, if you're a bit rusty!
- Bonus *free* idea: talking of the great outdoors, many council parks now have outdoor gyms with the kind of equipment you'd find in a traditional gym – but you get fresh air at the same time.

And *relax…*

OK, you're done! Time to relax… Do remember to keep a record of your week and to treat yourself well.

If at first you do find it a struggle, then keep going. It's taken me all my adult life to find a regime that suits me – and following the 5:2 Diet has certainly helped me, not to mention the research I've done for this book *and* the previous two.

What I've realised about myself is that I find exercise boring and repetitive. So my strategy has two strands – the gym, and micro-movements. I make the effort to move more in my work routine, and then at the gym, I focus my workouts on maximum intensity at the time, to maximise feeling virtuous after. I enjoy running now, thanks to Couch to 5K, but I also use the cross-trainer at the gym. I listen to BBC podcasts to counter the boredom. And I will never, ever be in a team again (unless it's a pub quiz). So my regime means I try to:

- do some intense exercise at least twice a week (ideally three times), at the gym, when it's as quiet as possible, so I can sweat and be as uncoordinated as I like with no one watching
- do some really basic work with hand weights after my workout and at home in front of the telly if I remember
- do 10,000 steps five days a week (I'll only feel disappointed if I aim for 7 days)
- get up and move around whenever I remember (and certainly when my Pomodairo tells me to!)
- **never feel guilty if I don't quite manage it one week because of illness or travel, for example – but simply get back to normal as soon as I can.**

As a result, I feel more confident about my body and my fitness. And if I can do it, I promise you can too!

Move Week: key points

Here's a summary of our key points from this week:

- Movement and flexibility is at least as important to our well-being as conventional gym-based exercise.
- Avoid being sedentary – move around at home and at work to ward off health problems.
- Begin small – committing yourself to small-scale targets, but with an objective and a way to monitor your progress.
- Vary what you do to avoid boredom and to keep challenging yourself.

Week 5

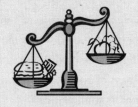

Nothing can bring you peace but yourself.

Ralph Waldo Emerson

Week 5: checking in

Before we get cracking on this week's theme, take a moment to review how you've felt about the Move experience!

- Have you managed to fit more NEAT-style micro-movements into your day? It won't take long for these to become a habit.

- Keep a record of how far you walked/ran/cycled or how far you could get into a workout video before running out of breath – so you keep track of how rapidly you're improving. And also make sure you note down how you feel before and after your activities?

- My top tip: use the information you're gathering to plan even better and more enjoyable sessions that challenge you without putting you off! I keep a record of the distance I travel and how long it takes me after each run. Beating your personal best is a great feeling.

Relax

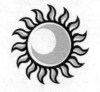

THIS WEEK'S AIM:
to relax fully, sleep well – and discover how good stress can
make your spare time more *satisfying and enjoyable*

Introduction

This week we're going to work on relaxation, 'spare' time – and sleep! 'Me-time' is an annoying phrase, but this is what we're looking at: making the most of precious time to do what you want and to recharge your batteries. It should be so simple – yet too often, sleep and relaxation are a struggle.

On Relax Day 1, we're focusing on rest and sleep – and what science can tell us about how to get the most from both. We'll explore simple techniques that can help us feel rested and restored (and have more energy when we need it!).

And on Relax Day 2, we're looking at 'spare' time – we'll look at how to make the most of leisure, discover why hobbies are good for us and explore how stress *can* be good for us – if we take control.

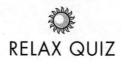

RELAX QUIZ

Make yourself a nice cuppa and relax with this laid-back mini quiz, to get you in the mood for this week's themes...

This week: **how you relax**

1   How do you sleep?

    A   Like a contented baby – at least 12 hours a night. I love my bed.

    B   Like a FTSE 100 executive – I only need 4 hours a night.

    C   Like a toddler – I can't sleep when I'm supposed to, and it makes me want to wail.

    D   It depends on what else is going on in my life. At times of stress, I find sleep harder but mostly it's OK and I can always catch up with naps during the day.

2   Where do you keep your mobile phone at night?

    A   Wherever I left it – in my bag or the living room.

    B   On the bedside table, or even under the duvet, in case Seattle calls or I get an urgent Tweet to respond to.

    C   In the bedroom, even though it keeps me awake at night with the lights, but I'm worried someone might call in an emergency. Plus, I can play games if insomnia strikes.

    D   In the bedroom, but only because I use it as an alarm clock.

3   What's your average stress level, on a scale of 1 to 10?
    A   2 or 3. I don't really get stressed about anything.
    B   Pretty high – 7 or 8. But I like stress, most of the
         time – it helps me feel alive!
    C   10. I rarely relax but if you had my life, you'd be
         the same.
    D   It varies hugely. I do get stressed when bad things
         happen, but I don't dwell on it for too long.

If you found yourself drawn to…

Mostly As: you are gloriously relaxed and well rested. But if occasionally you might want to be less of a dormouse, this week will show why the odd bit of controlled stress is no bad thing.

Mostly Bs: you seem to thrive on pressure, but there could be long-term consequences if you never chill out. Speed-read your way through this week to find out how slowing down could be a good thing, now and then.

Mostly Cs: life might seem out of control for you at the moment, but there are some really simple techniques and ideas that might relieve those feelings of pressure. Try to make just a little time to focus on this week's activities.

Mostly Ds: You're an example to us all! You've worked out that your attitude to stress is as important as the stress itself. This week's activities will put that attitude into context and help you keep calm and carry on…

RELAX DAY 1: REST

Sleep…

It's one of my favourite occupations!

But for something so natural and essential, sleep can be a troublesome and elusive thing. Even quite low-level disruptions to sleep patterns – like jet lag or a partner's snoring – can leave you feeling wrecked.

So, today we're going to look at the essentials of good sleep, and also think about how we can find other ways and times to relax and rest. We'll explore meditation and mindfulness as techniques to help (don't worry, there are no lotus positions involved) and how turning off electronic 'chatter' can help your body turn off properly too.

5:2 INSPIRATIONS

WHAT IS SLEEP?

According to good old Wikipedia, sleep is a 'naturally recurring state characterised by reduced or absent consciousness, relatively suspended sensory activity, and inactivity of nearly all voluntary muscles.'

There are four stages to the sleep 'cycle' and the body progresses through them every time we fall asleep. REM sleep – the stage when our eyes move rapidly, and when we usually dream – comes last. We spend around 20–25% of our sleep time in that mode, though if we wake too soon we may not reach that stage. (To read more about the stages, try en.wikipedia.org/wiki/Sleep)

But *why* do we need to sleep at all? Despite extensive research and many dedicated sleep labs around the world, scientists are not 100% sure... One theory is that sleep conserves energy, yet studies show we only use perhaps 5–10% less energy during sleeping hours than when we're awake. A related idea is that it's about safety – that feeling tired may protect many animals, including humans, from the potential dangers of being active in the dark/at night.

Another theory that's gaining more attention is the idea that REM sleep helps us manage difficult emotional experiences. During that phase, experiences are processed while chemicals that relate to stress, like norepinephrine, are suppressed, potentially helping us to gain distance and reduce the emotional impact caused by difficult experiences.

A different, but intriguing, idea focuses on the glymphatic system which helps remove waste products from the brain. One team of researchers has identified this system as being more active in mice when they're asleep. If further research shows the same in humans, it may demonstrate that sleep has a 'housekeeping' function which may reduce the build-up of damaged proteins which are often seen in patients with diseases including Alzheimer's and Parkinson's. This may mirror some of the housekeeping done by the body during fasting, which is one of the key benefits of 5:2.

As research continues, no doubt even more theories will emerge, but here's what we do know about the impact of sleep (or the lack of it) on the body:

- Immune systems – sleep deprivation has been shown to lower the number of infection-fighting white blood cells in animals.
- It may also reduce the build-up of free radicals in the brain, which cause cell damage.
- Healing – studies suggest that the rate of healing of wounds may be slower if we're sleep deprived.
- Memory – working memory, the kind we use for everyday tasks (also sometimes called short-term memory), is definitely reduced by too little sleep, affecting our ability to learn, problem-solve and pay attention.
- Development in children – newborn babies need up to 18 hours of sleep a day, and REM sleep appears to help brain development.
- Death rates – see the next section but people who get the 'right' amount of sleep seem to live longer than those who get too little or too much.

How much is just right?

There's no easy answer to this question because, like the three bears and their porridge portions, the amount of sleep we need varies from person to person. The age we are is an important element, though genetics are also likely to play a part.

Certainly, children need more sleep than grown-ups, but for adults the suggested guideline is 7–9 hours a night. Many studies have shown that people who have significantly less sleep, and conversely, people who have significantly more sleep, have lower life expectancies. It's hard to separate out cause and effect. So people who sleep more or less than usual may have other medical complications, which could affect their sleep. But good health and good sleep are connected.

When to sleep? Naps and siestas

Sleep doesn't have to be all in one go – taking naps or siestas may offer health benefits, especially when it comes to the heart and blood pressure.

Regularly taking a siesta is associated with a 37% drop in death from heart diseases. As always, it's hard to pinpoint the reasons, but at least one study suggests that the reduction in blood pressure as your body prepares for and starts to sleep could be a really important factor. Even anticipating a nap may help lower your blood pressure.

The sleep debt, insomnia and other sleep disorders

Just as having too little money to meet our needs drains our bank balance, having too little sleep drains our energy reserves and causes strain to the body. Sleep debt builds, so that over time, our mental and physical functioning deteriorates. We can catch up at weekends, but that in itself can upset the balance and rhythm of regular sleep patterns. For something that appears so natural, sleep can be a sensitive thing.

Extended sleep deprivation or debt may be linked to the following:

- cardiovascular problems including heart disease, heart attack, high blood pressure and stroke
- Type 2 diabetes
- higher risk of accidents
- poor concentration
- weight gain
- depression.

5:2 MYTH-BUSTING

WHY COUNTING SHEEP DOESN'T WORK

I remember trying the sheep-counting idea as a teenager. I don't remember it working very well; I kept inventing different outfits for the sheep and making them fall over the stile to relieve the monotony – and now scientists at Oxford University have proved me right. It's too boring to work for most of us, whereas picturing a relaxing scene, like a beach or beautiful countryside, helped insomniacs in the study fall asleep on average 20 minutes faster than the sheep did.

Improving your zzzzz

If you're an insomniac, it's pretty frustrating to read about the dangers of the 'wrong kind of sleep'. But the good news is that there are many steps we can take to improve sleep quality. And if you already sleep well, and feel rested, then well done! But you can still enhance your quality of relaxation with the activity and the challenge that follow.

Sleep hygiene

No, this doesn't mean that you need to have a shower or floss your teeth before hitting the sack. It's about setting up patterns of behaviour and making changes to your environment that maximise your chances of getting the most from your rest time.

Today's bonus activity will take you through a programme to ensure you're doing everything you can to maximise your chances of sleeping or relaxing. But before that we're going to look at how meditation can benefit all of us, whether we sleep like babies, or rarely sleep at all.

Meditation, mindfulness and what it all means

All together now… Ommm.

Only kidding. Meditation means different things to different people, and that can be a problem. For some of us, the word conjures up tie-dye kaftans, facial hair and uncomfortable yoga positions, and that's enough to put many people off.

The kind of meditation we're going to focus on is free of religious or 'hippie' philosophy. There are no mantras needed, or special clothes. I was sceptical at first, but now I'd describe mindfulness meditation as being a short break from the stresses of work or home life. It involves taking a little time to check how we're feeling and what's happening in the body, and trying to accept and focus on being aware of the present, rather than dwelling on the past or worrying about the future.

Though 'mindfulness' meditation does contain elements of Buddhist practice, you don't need to have any particular beliefs to try it. You simply need a little time, and a chair.

WHAT MINDFULNESS MEDITATION CAN DO

In 2013, researchers brought together 200 different studies on the use of Mindfulness Based Therapy (MBT) for conditions including anxiety, stress and depression. The studies had involved over 12,000 patients, and the overall conclusion was that it could be a very effective treatment for psychological issues. Insomnia is another problem that can be reduced through meditation, improving sleep but also minimising the stress sleeplessness can cause.

I am not making any claims as a meditation guru and I don't own any robes or have any diplomas – but I have tried different techniques, and found they've made me feel calmer and better able to deal with stress.

Key Activity, Relax Day 1
meditation's what you need

I'm offering two different options here: either a very simple version of mindfulness or a choice of websites, apps or books offering more detailed guidance and guided downloads, which you may find easier.

Whichever appeals most, I *do* urge you to try it, even if you're a little cynical. I promise, there's nothing to lose and potentially a lot to gain!

Option A Self-guided mindfulness

Step 1: the place

Find a place where you can be still and feel safe…

It could be an upright chair, or a cushion on the floor with your back resting against the wall or some furniture, but nothing on wheels – it needs to be somewhere that you can sit down, distraction-free, and then pretty much forget you are there.

You could imagine that you've found a place in the forest, with your back against a sturdy oak. Or that you're in a beachside cove, seated with sun-warmed rock supporting your back.

Sit down, with your hands on your thighs and your back straight. You should be relaxed and not rigid.

Feel your own body in the space: your feet or legs resting on the floor, your hands on your legs, your back supported.

You don't have to close your eyes yet. Just let your focus soften, as though you don't want to focus on anything in particular but simply accept everything that's in the room around you.

Stay as you are for a while… there's no rush. You're not thinking about the past, or the future, only this moment, sitting in a safe place.

Your mind *will* wander. Don't worry. Gently bring yourself back to where you are now, to the feeling of your body making contact with the floor, or the chair, and the present.

Step 2: the breath

Begin to notice your breathing.

Don't try to alter it now. Simply be aware of the in-breath entering your body, and the out-breath leaving. It's a cycle we take for granted but it's at the heart of everything our body does.

Your breath may slow a little as you become more conscious of it. Or it may not. Don't judge, or worry. Mindfulness is about observing and accepting.

When it feels natural to do so, close your eyes.

Step 3: the body

Begin to notice how your body feels. Start at your toes and slowly scan up your body mentally, taking time to notice how each part of you is feeling. Do this in an unhurried way: from your toes, to your feet, the muscles in your lower legs, your thighs. Be aware of how your skin feels, any heaviness where your body is in contact with the chair or floor.

If you sense any discomfort or pain, observe it without trying to change it. Accept it and then move onto the next part of the body. If you feel tension, focus back on your breathing for a few moments.

Continue scanning through the hips, the torso, the chest: be aware that your internal organs are working, too, to keep your body functioning. Notice your hands, your arms, back, shoulders and neck. If there is any tension, acknowledge it and move on.

Finally, the head and face. Be aware of your skin, mouth, nose, eyes. Notice your in-breath and out-breath: move the scan to the forehead, up to the top of the head.

Now notice your body as a whole. Feel how the breath is giving life to your body as you sit.

Step 4: the mind

As you let your mind be calm, and focus on place, then breath, then body, your thoughts *will* wander. Acknowledge this, and slowly and gently bring your focus back to the present: to the breath, and the body.

After you've completed the body scan, you can gradually begin to bring your attention back to your surroundings.

When you feel ready, open your eyes.

Take a minute or two to notice your breathing and how this time out has made you feel.

A note on timing: to begin with, you can aim for 10 minutes, but as time goes by, you can increase the time to suit you.

Option B Audio/download options

Many of us will find it easier to follow a meditation we can listen to. I've provided more sites in the resources section in Part Four on page 352 or alternatively, you could record the meditation yourself on your phone or computer and listen back to it when you need to.

Key Activity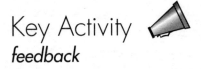
feedback

How was that for you?

When I first tried mindfulness, it was much simpler than I expected – no chanting, no special language. I did wonder at first what all the fuss was about, and at the beginning I found it hard to stay on track; even now, I get days when it's easier than others. But there's something about the moments of mindfulness that I find addictive in the best way – it's energising and de-stressing and takes very little time out of the day.

How often should you meditate?

At a minimum, try meditation twice this week, on your 5:2 days. But as today's activity only lasted around 10 minutes instead of the usual 30, perhaps you can try meditating more than twice? As with a small number of other activities in this book – including Worry o'clock and expressive writing – there can be additional benefits if you are able to carve out a little time most days. It could become a healthy 'addiction' you decide to embrace after the 5:2 Your Life plan is over.

A less healthy addiction: the dangers of cyber-chatter...

Let me start this next part with an admission: if there's one bad habit I have yet to crack, it's this one.

I've never been a smoker (well, apart from a few fags in a vain attempt to look cool when I should have known better) but I reckon the internet is as addictive as nicotine. And, of course, it's still socially acceptable and allowed in pubs and public places.

A few years ago, the big worry was that mobile signals would fry the brain. Now, my big worry is that social networking might fry the attention span. E-chatter is, for me, the total opposite of mindfulness. The demands and status updates, emails, blogs and online data are constant and almost infinite.

Some scary stats

Here are some scary statistics on internet use (mostly found on the internet, of course!):

- In Britain, web users spend one in every 12 waking minutes online – that's about 90 minutes per day – some surveys suggest it's even higher, as much as 4 hours per day.
- 62% of us reach for our smartphones before we do anything else in the morning.
- 51% of us feel extreme anxiety if separated from our phones.

And it's getting harder to escape the tyrant in your pocket – it's even more annoying if your companion is busily checking emails between courses in a restaurant, or tweeting from that gig or performance rather than embracing the moment.

In addition to the everyday irritations, some scientists believe that constantly updating our status and refreshing our emails may have longer-term effects on the brain, potentially reducing our concentration span. We may become both more self-obsessed *and* less confident, as we constantly compare ourselves to others.

Stopping the cyber-rot, 007-style

It doesn't have to be that way. I'm not suggesting you throw the BlackBerry out with the bathwater, but in true 5:2 style, the best way to change unproductive habits is to start small, and make a choice to reduce the constant presence of those smartphones and tablets.

According to the newspapers, James Bond actor Daniel Craig and his wife, Rachel Weisz, believe the secret of a happy marriage is to ban technology from the bedroom… In September 2013, the *Daily Telegraph* quoted him as saying, 'there's nothing technological allowed in the bedroom. If the iPad goes to bed, I mean, unless you're watching porn on the internet, it's a killer. We have a ban on it.'

Leaving aside what 007 has on his iPad, I think what's good for Hollywood stars could be good for you too. If you ban technology, you'll also be getting rid of annoying electronic noises, strange lights glowing in the middle of the night and even that sense of being on call 24/7. So let's try out a challenge that's worthy of James Bond.

Challenge, Relax Day 1
cyber-detox

This is possibly the simplest challenge yet.

Tonight, go to bed without your smartphone or your iPad or your MP3 player. In fact, remove all electronic devices from the bedroom – if you have a TV, switch it off at the mains. A clock radio is borderline, but try to do without it. Otherwise, *nothing else*.

To deal with a few practicalities, if you use your phone as an alarm, put it just beyond the bedroom door (that snooze button is a waste of time anyway: one study suggests Britons waste almost 85 hours per year by hitting snooze each morning). Or find an old clockwork alarm clock. If you're a heart surgeon on call, you can leave the phone within reach, but turn off all other functions.

If you don't normally go to sleep straight away, read a book, or try mindfulness. Or, if you share a bed, well, you know…

When you wake up in the morning, stretch out your limbs and take five long, deep breaths, before checking your emails. Once you're used to that, try delaying that first email/Twitter check until you reach work.

If you're struggling, write down how you're feeling about being offline. Are you anxious about missing out? Ask yourself what the likelihood is that you'll miss something urgent while you're asleep…

Extending the detox

Once you've tried that first night without technology, push yourself a little further. Leave your phone at home or in airplane mode when you go out with your partner or friends. Keep it out of sight at dinner. And if you *must* view YouTube videos in the evening, watch them alongside the person you're sharing the sofa with… they might enjoy them too!

What if my bedroom – and life – is already a zen, cyber-chatter free zone?

You're entitled to feel very smug. Your challenge today is to look at your pleasure list (if you have one) and choose something nice to reward yourself for your all-round goodness! If you don't have a list, start one!

Challenge: feedback

Was that harder than you thought – or a breath of fresh air?

I'm not trying to be holier than thou and this is not about turning back the clock to a pre-internet age or denying that technology can bring many benefits – it's simply about carving out time for human interaction and simpler, more restful pursuits.

And, in the process, I bet you get a better night's sleep…

Speaking of which:

Bonus Activity, Relax Day 1
the big sleep makeover

Hopefully you've seen how a small difference – like banning technology from the bedroom – can change the atmosphere completely.

This activity builds on the science of 'sleep hygiene' (see page 190) to maximise your chances of a great night's sleep.

Not all the ideas will necessarily apply to you, so work your way through from a to zzzzz…

Step 1: Setting the scene
Is your bedroom as sleep-friendly as possible? Think about:
- **Light:** can you reduce any light from streetlamps, or daylight if you're a shift worker? Blackout blinds can be

cheap and easily fitted and work well behind curtains (they can reduce heating bills in winter too).

- **Noise:** you may have limited control over this if there are external sources of noise, but earplugs are worth trying. If you need an alarm clock, then daylight alarm clocks which simulate sunrise to wake you can be an alternative to ones which beep!
- **Scents/air:** it's hard to sleep in a stuffy room so try opening the window to air the space for a while before you go to bed. Aromatherapy oil diffusers can help to make you feel more relaxed – lavender is a favourite of mine. Or buy a pillow spray for soothing scents when you go to sleep.
- **Temperature:** you'll struggle to sleep if you're too hot or too cold. It's best to keep the bedroom at a slightly cooler temperature than the rest of the house.
- **Bedding:** this is also a factor in how hot/cold you're going to feel, so make sure you've got the right bedding for the season. If you can, treat yourself to a new set of bedding or pillows or something new to wear in bed – it's a worthwhile investment when you think how much time you spend there!
- **Technology:** don't forget to cut it right down or eliminate it all together (see the 007 challenge earlier!).

Step 2: Preparing your body for sleep

Your routine before you go to bed plays an important part in how well you'll sleep, so think about establishing good rituals:

- **Food:** try to avoid heavy meals immediately before bed – though a light snack can be worth trying. Cheese and bananas contain tryptophan which can help with sleep – kiwi fruits and cherries may also help.

- **Drink:** too much alcohol can lead to sleepless nights – it may help you fall asleep but as levels in the blood drop, you may well wake up again during the night. Most of us avoid coffee before bed but tea also contains caffeine so herbal teas can be a better idea. A milky drink can encourage sleep and some stores sell pints from cows milked early in the morning, when their levels of melatonin are at their highest. The hormone is linked to the regulation of our body clocks (known as circadian rhythms) though the exact effects are unclear.
- **Exercising** during the day can be beneficial but not in the two to three hours immediately before you go to bed. Also avoid scary or over-stimulating TV or video games.
- **A warm bath** or shower using relaxing scents can 'prepare' your mind and body for sleep.
- **Time:** keeping to roughly the same bedtime and wake-up time during weekdays and weekends means the body gets used to sleep times. Napping on and off during the day is better avoided, though an afternoon siesta that lasts no longer than 30–45 minutes can be beneficial.

Step 3: Calming the mind

- Leave your worries outside the bedroom. I know it's easier said than done, but you could write down what you need to do tomorrow before settling down to bed, so you know it's safely recorded and there's no risk of forgetting.
- Try mindfulness to accept those thoughts – or relaxation/ sleep CDs or MP3s to guide you towards sleep (the only technological option allowed!).
- Reading is a low-tech way to relax and stop you fixating on worries or issues.

Step 4: In case of (sleep) emergency...

- If at first you don't succeed... stop trying. Seriously, this is often the hardest advice to follow, but the longer you stay awake, fretting about not being able to sleep, the more risk there is of a negative pattern becoming established.
- If you haven't fallen asleep within 30 minutes of trying and feel anxious, get out of bed and go to another room. Don't turn the telly or laptop on – the light can fool your body into thinking it's morning – read instead or try a bath or a small snack.
- Try going back to bed after 20–30 minutes, but if you still can't sleep and are feeling stressed, then get up again. Keep everything low-key, including your own feelings about sleep – the less wound up you are, the more likely you are to be able to sleep eventually.
- Change your routine... if you struggle to sleep on a particular night of the week – Sunday is pretty common – then do something quite different, like going out on the town rather than going to bed early and then fretting. You could even embrace the insomnia and give yourself permission to stay awake all night if you can't sleep – it's a version of the stimulus control idea in the Worry o' clock exercise in Week 1 (see page 41).
- If you're struggling over a longer period of days or weeks, talk to your doctor – various medical conditions and prescription drugs can affect sleep patterns, so do take their advice. It doesn't have to mean taking medication for sleep issues, but sometimes that can be a short-term aid.

For more hints and detail, go to the University of Maryland Medical Center page, via this link, http://bit.ly/1h5EVv5.

Zzzz…

I think that's enough for Day 1… we'll be looking at reducing bad stress and maximising fun on Day 2. In the meantime, sweet dreams…

RELAX DAY 2: AT EASE

You know that song… 'Easy like Sunday morning'?

Let's set aside for a moment the fact that the *lyrics* are actually about some bloke making excuses for leaving his girlfriend. For me, the *melody* suggests the very best kind of Sunday morning, the whole day ahead, feeling mellow, not much planned but so many enticing possibilities…

But how many Sunday mornings *are* like that? Too often there's urgent DIY to be finished, the back garden's in a state, you have demanding visitors, the shopping needs doing, and the kids need nagging to do homework, plus really you should be catching up with emails and bills and…

I can feel the stress levels rising just *writing* about it!

So let's take a minute to talk about stress… because it's not all bad – so long as it's the right *kind* of stress.

What is stress?

At its simplest, stress is our response to stuff that happens to us. Usually, when we talk about stress, we mean an unpleasant physical response. That might be a temporary response like a rapid heartbeat or a headache due to a work deadline or an argument. Or it might be longer-term symptoms like anxiety, insomnia, depression or high blood pressure, triggered by a problem like unemployment or divorce.

The idea of seeing stress as an undesirable response to circumstances is less than a hundred years old – it was first described in the 1920s. But the physical response we experience is ancient: our early ancestors would have experienced similar 'fight or flight' responses to physical dangers. This includes the release of hormones including epinephrine (also known as adrenalin), which helps to regulate blood flow so we have more energy to respond to danger, and of cortisol, which boosts blood sugar to help us act and think faster.

How does that sound so far? Maybe I'm weird, but I actually quite *like* the idea of acting and thinking faster…

Good stress vs bad stress

So is it possible to *enjoy* stress? I think I do. I like trying new things. I like scary movies and TV (well, scary-ish – I draw the line at *The Walking Dead*). To my surprise, I even like running, a form of physical stress that pushes my heart rate and breathing to the max. I almost always find I can do more than I thought I'd manage before I started the run.

I believe *good* stress – pushing yourself – can help you to enjoy your spare time. Whether it's the adrenalin-crazed stress of a hill climb, or the mental stress of a tricky Sudoku, we feel better when we set ourselves a challenge. Even if we don't *quite* achieve it, we learn from it, and do it better next time! Stress that we actively choose to experience can make us feel alive.

The problem comes when stress is constant – and out of our control.

Stress – or strain?

Engineers define stress as when a piece of equipment has to work hard but within its capability. Strain is when the machine is being pushed too far. The equipment may suffer damage, or work less efficiently.

That's what happens to us when the stressors in our lives are too severe or too constant. Hormones like cortisol and epinephrine that are designed to provide a short-term fix can have damaging effects if they're in our systems all the time. We feel bad – jittery, anxious, depressed – and can gain weight, suffer digestive issues, feel tired all the time, even suffer chest pains.

One solution is to try to find ways of minimising the day-to-day stressors, or to minimise their effects using techniques that make us feel under control. We already encountered some useful methods, like the Pomodoro Technique (see page 53) to Worry o'clock (see page 41).

It also seems that one of the keys to managing stress *might* be simply to stop stressing about it so much in the first place.

5:2 INSPIRATIONS

RETHINKING STRESS

In a great example of the Puppy Effect (see page 58), a wonderful TED video was released just as I was beginning to put together this section on stress. If you haven't come across TED (Technology, Entertainment, Design), it's a great site (with apps for your tablet or smartphone) featuring inspiring talks by fantastic speakers from all backgrounds.

This particular talk, (available at bit.ly/1jbml16) by psychologist Kelly McGonigal, echoed my own feelings about stress, and it's definitely worth watching. Her research suggests it may not be stress in itself that's damaging. It may be simply whether we *view* stress as damaging!

McGonigal recaps on the physical effects of serious stress – including how it can make our blood vessels constrict temporarily, which could increase our risk of cardiovascular diseases. Then she describes a study in which students were trained to view the 'fight or flight' responses (for example, an increase in heart rate or breathing) as positive preparation for a challenging situation. So the pounding heart shows your body is becoming energised and preparing for action, and the faster breathing helps more oxygen get to the brain to figure out the best way to deal with a situation.

When those students with a positive view of stress were monitored, their blood vessels *didn't* narrow – their responses were heightened but their physical sensations appeared much **more like joy and less like fear** or panic.

Other studies showed that where people had experienced severe stress *and thought it would damage their health*, they had a 30% increase in the risk of premature death per stressful event (and we're talking serious stress like death of a family member or losing your job or home). Yet when individuals didn't believe stress would damage their health, there was no increased risk of death.

This may not be the whole story: the effect that stress or anger and our basic personality have on heart health is complex so these studies aren't conclusive. But it does make sense that finding a way to accept stress – the same way mindfulness helps you notice how the body is feeling without trying to change it – could be beneficial.

Stress – and the 'cuddle hormone'

Remember from the Connect chapter how helping others can make you happy? McGonigal presents additional evidence that caring may also counteract stress.

The study on deaths following stressful events, indicated that people who spent some of their time caring for others showed no increase in risk of death at all! McGonigal believes this is partly thanks to oxytocin. Oxytocin has been nicknamed the 'cuddle hormone' because it encourages us to seek physical contact with others. But it also helps counteract the 'stressing' effect of fight or flight hormones. It reduces damaging inflammation and can even help the heart regenerate.

In fact, it may not even have to be *people* you're caring for – one research study from Japan showed pet owners who played with their dogs and looked them in the eye during play showed a 20% increase in oxytocin readings.

Working out what we want

Right at the end of that video, McGonigal says: 'Chasing meaning is better for your health than trying to avoid discomfort.'

I don't talk much about spirituality in this book, but most of us do want to find meaning in our lives. That search can be uncomfortable, even painful. But it's not a reason to stop. It *is* a reason to nurture yourself as well as others.

Right now we're going to take an overview of your life, and how you balance your many roles, duties and dreams.

Key Activity 1, Relax Day 2
the 5:2 ferris wheel of life (or the 5:2 pie)

Is your life in apple pie order... or do you have too many fingers in too many pies? We're going to draw a ferris wheel – or a pie – to find out.

This activity builds on what you did in Week 1, and is adapted from an exercise in *The Artist's Way* book by Julia Cameron. It gives you a snapshot of how things are right now, and it's easy to repeat further down the line to check your progress!

Step 1: list all the roles you play in life
These might include family roles, jobs, hobbies and ambitions. Think about the different ways you spend both weekdays *and* weekends. You might be a:
- parent
- wife/husband/partner
- worker (e.g. doctor, teacher, secretary, builder, musician, carer)
- daughter/sister/son/brother
- friend
- grandparent/uncle/aunt/godparent
- cleaner/cook/domestic god or goddess

- household PA (organiser, chauffeur, holiday booker, gift buyer)
- photographer/singer/artist
- volunteer/fund-raiser/community rep/worshipper
- runner/footballer/swimmer/cyclist?

Step 2: draw your pie or wheel

- Now choose eight of these roles: include the ones you are committed to currently – like wife/husband, parent, worker – plus at least two that represent the things you enjoy most or want to do.
- Draw a circle and then divide it into eight like this: (or use the download available on the website)

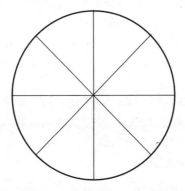

- Write each role outside the circle, where each line meets the outside edge. Now place a dot on each straight line depending on how well you feel you're playing that role. If it's going perfectly, place the dot right on the outer edge. If you feel you're neglecting it, or unable to spend enough time on it, place the dot nearer the centre (see my example to make it clearer).

- Now draw a line linking each of the dots.

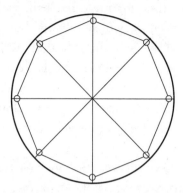

Step 3: how does your pie or wheel look?

- Look at your pie or wheel. In an ideal world, it would look like this – just like the London Eye or a very neat open-topped pie.
- Chances are, it won't look anything like that. But it will help you see how you might change the way you slice up your life.

As an example, this is how my wheel/pie looks right now:

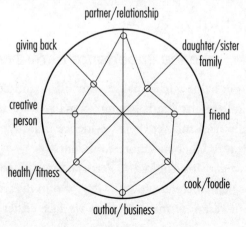

As you can see, my life isn't perfectly balanced – I'm doing pretty well with time for my other half, with cooking (lots of recipe testing lately, which is work but also a passion), and writing and keeping fit/a healthy weight. But work commitments have knocked me off balance in other roles, and I want to spend more time with family and friends, and to nurture my creative side by making some clothes and starting my next novel. So, once I've finished editing *this* book, I know what to do!

Now it's over to you! Look at where your graph looks out of balance – for many of us, it's the enjoyable elements that we tend to neglect.

Step 4: re-balance your roles

Pick the role that you're neglecting and choose something you can do today – or this week – to nurture that side of you and your dreams. The key is not to feel guilty about any areas that are off-balance right now, but to use the activity to help you plan to put that right!

Key Activity

feedback – and the importance of resilience

The wheel/pie helps you visualise your life – and competing demands. You might think having so many roles to fulfil is automatically stressful. Yet there's evidence that juggling roles can make you tougher and more confident.

Yale University psychologist, Patricia Linville, found that the more 'layers' there are to our view of ourselves, the more balanced our response may be when we face either hardship or good times. If we see ourselves as many-faceted, we're less likely to feel destroyed if one part of our life is going badly… At the same time, if we have a big success in one area, we're still realistic about ourselves as a 'whole' person – we don't let it go to our heads!

Resilience – the ability to cope with adversity and stress – sounds like something that is built in, that you either have or don't have, yet we can work on building it. Factors that can increase resilience include:

- having a strong network of friends or family
- having high levels of self-esteem
- setting goals for yourself
- tackling problems rather than letting them get worse
- having a sense of purpose.

So, finding activities and hobbies you enjoy and feel you're good at, isn't just about fun – it can also make you tougher!

'Role play' – finding free time for fun

Do you feel you have no free time to pursue your different roles?

Maybe you could try turning off the TV? The average British person spends 4 hours 2 minutes daily watching television (though, of course, we often combine TV watching with other activities, like eating or doing admin).

And what about the thorny question of who has more free time – men or women? The Organisation for Economic Co-operation and Development (OECD)– which studies nations including the UK, US, Australia and European countries – says British women tend to have 32 minutes less leisure time than men, but they spend 22 minutes more than the guys on personal care like bathing… (maybe switching to a shower will give you more time to have fun!)

Internationally:

The average person in the OECD works 1, 776 hours a year and devotes 62% of the day, or close to 15 hours, to personal care (eating, sleeping, etc.) and leisure (socializing with friends and family, hobbies, games, computer and television use, etc.).

You can compare notes at oecdbetterlifeindex.org – but how will *you* spend *your* free hours? TV and the internet have their place, but they're passive. For our challenge today, we're stepping up – and away from the screen!

Challenge, Relax Day 2
get real!

Yes, those screens can be mesmerising – but many activities are simply more fun in the real world than online. So this challenge is about rediscovering the enjoyment to be had from sharing your passions and interests.

Step 1
Write a list of things you do at home or online – choose fun stuff you do as part of your routine or in your leisure time, for example:

1 Singing in the shower/dancing in the kitchen/watching *Strictly Come Dancing*.

2   Taking photographs with my phone and uploading them onto the net.
3   Watch the football on TV.
4   Doing an exercise video.
5   Researching holiday destinations or places to visit.
6   Knitting, sewing or dress-making.
7   Learning a language using an app or online videos.
8   Trying new recipes (and trying not to eat all the leftovers).

Step 2

Brainstorm 'real world' equivalents... think about how you could use your passions to be more active and connected.

1   Join a choir or a salsa or tango class (most organise trial sessions before you have to commit full time).
2   Try a photography safari or class.
3   Go to the pub to watch the football with a local supporters' group – or even buy a ticket for the stadium.
4   Join an exercise class or organised walk.
5   Go to the library and look at the magazines, guide and photography books or leaflets.
6   Find a 'stitch and bitch' group near you – or set one up.
7   Find a language exchange/intercambio where native speakers and local speakers take turns to try conversation.
8   Join the Clandestine Cake Club (which meets up to make different themed cakes, with branches across the UK) or a supper club where you share dishes in each other's homes.

Step 3

Choose the one that appeals the most and arrange to do it this week – or as soon as possible! It doesn't even have to cost money. One great online research for real-world activities is www.meetup.com where people set up clubs or groups for an amazing range of interests.

I just checked upcoming events in my area and they included free yoga, a Winnie-the-Pooh walk, a 'one hour, six pictures' event for photographers, climbing lessons and a 'gig buddies' group for people wanting to see bands without having to go on their own!

It's the perfect place to look to help you find an event or hobby that fits the bill for your bonus activity...

Bonus Activity, Relax Day 2
do something scary!

I want you to do something scary, or stressful – or both.

This is your chance to put the ideas about stress into practice and learn to love the feeling of pushing yourself.

Step 1
Brainstorm some ideas for raising your heartbeat in a scarily enjoyable way:

- **Heights:** monkey rope/jungle adventure park, climbing wall at local leisure centre, London Eye, a rollercoaster.
- **Fears for fun:** a scary late-night movie screening, a suspenseful theatre performance, a ghost walk...
- **Competition:** try a quiz night, bowling, a treasure hunt.
- **Spontaneity/adventure:** go to the train or bus station and get on the first bus or train (buy a ticket first!), try a

new kind of food, go to a shop you've never visited, buy clothes you'd usually avoid (I tried jeggings for the first time this year – a cross between leggings and jeans – and never looked back!), book a speed-dating night.

Alternatively... go the other way:
- if your life is already packed with adventure, try the opposite by choosing to have an hour where you do nothing except stare out of the window or read a book! That can be scary if you're a frantic kind of person.
- Or if you suffer from information overload, try a reading ban for a day (an idea from *The Artist's Way*) – avoid media and books and focus on the natural world instead.

Step 2
Do one of these!

Step 3
Jot down notes about how your choice made you feel before, during and afterwards. Did the fear or unfamiliarity energise you, make you see the world differently?

Keep your list and add to it, whenever you feel like shaking up your routine.

Relax Week: key points
Here's a summary of our key points from this week:
- Sleep – establishing good routines will help you find the quality and quantity of sleep that suits your body's needs.
- Meditation is simple and can be beneficial whatever your spiritual outlook or your lifestyle. It can take as little as 10 minutes.

- Switching off technology helps you switch off the brain…
- But a little stress can be good for you and even good fun, so long as you feel in control of intensity.

Week 6

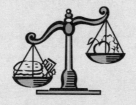

*The two most important days
in your life are the day you
are born and the day
you find out why.*

Mark Twain

Week 6: checking in

How has your week been since your last 5:2 day?

- Have you worked on your sleep routine? Try not to make bedtime a source of anxiety!

- How did the meditation go? If you're enjoying it, don't restrict yourself to the two 5:2 days – you can enjoy a spot of me-time whenever it suits you. I even did a mini-meditation in the post office queue today.

- Have you tried something scary but enjoyable? If not, why not recruit a friend to team up with so you can challenge each other to new heights of bravery?

Do!

THIS WEEK'S AIM:
to work out what you're best at – and how to do more of it.

Introduction

It's our final week – and we're getting to work on what we do and how we make a difference. We're not simply looking at paid jobs, but how we can use our passions and our talents in all aspects of life. We're also reviewing how we can keep up the momentum once the 5:2 Your Life plan is over!

So on Do! Day 1 we'll explore how to get the right balance between what we *love* to do and what we *have* to do to pay the bills.

And on Do! Day 2, we'll celebrate what you've achieved in the last six weeks, and plan for doing even bigger and better things in future.

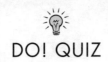

DO! QUIZ

Final week, final quiz. You know the score…
This week: **what you do!**

1   If you're working at the moment, how would you feel if
    someone offered you redundancy from your job, with a
    decent pay-off?

    A   Horrified – I love my job and would never give it
    up. I'd be anxious that they're even considering
    they could do without me.

    B   Unsure – I'd weigh it up with my partner and family.
    I like my job, but I could find another one, and the
    bonus money would be nice.

    C   Not keen – I prefer the security of my job, even if it
    bores me sometimes.

    D   Excited – I'd jump at it, to have the chance to
    retrain, set up my own business or go travelling.

2   You meet some new people on holiday and that question
    crops up: 'and what do *you* do?' What's your response?

    A   I was the one who asked the question – I think it
    tells you a lot when you find out how people spend
    most of their working hours. And I love talking about
    my work, whether it's paid or voluntary, or in the
    home.

    B   I tell them, but I'm more interested in finding out
    about them.

    C   I groan and try to change the subject. I'm on
    holiday and talking about work – or explaining why

I'm not in paid work – is almost as dull as being there.

D I wish they hadn't asked – my current job doesn't really reflect my personality or aspirations. So I talk about my future plans instead.

3 Have you made any retirement plans yet?

A I don't plan to retire completely – I'd like to go freelance and would miss the stimulation of work. Or I'd volunteer in the same field.

B Not really. I'll see how it goes but definitely want more time with friends and family.

C I started planning my retirement almost as soon as I started work. I hope to have a good, long time to do what I like, without my boss breathing down my neck.

D Retirement sounds boring. So long as I have enough money to stay afloat, I'm going to keep trying new things. It keeps you young!

If you found yourself drawn to…

Mostly As: others might describe you as a workaholic, but you don't care – your job gives you so much satisfaction. This week won't change that, but it might give you ideas to make your work even better.

Mostly Bs: you enjoy what you do, but don't want it to get in the way of the rest of your life. This week will give you ideas for making the most of what you do at work and at home, without upsetting the balance you work hard to achieve.

223

Mostly Cs: your work simply isn't the most important thing about you. But wouldn't it be nice to get a little more satisfaction out of that aspect of your life? Read on to discover how.

Mostly Ds: why have one career, when you can have three? Or six? You're someone who doesn't put up with things you don't like, which can be positive – but this week will help you focus on finding occupations that will keep you interested for as long as possible!

DO! DAY 1
A SENSE OF PURPOSE

And what do you do?

It's the big question that crops up at parties, on holiday or whenever you meet new people.

How does it make *you* feel? Excited to share the work you do because you love it and it makes a difference – or fearful that someone will judge you for your occupation, or because you aren't currently in paid work?

If we're lucky, the way we spend our working – or working from home – hours reflects our passions and talents and choices we've made. But often it's more about stuff that's happened to us: circumstances and commitments and caring responsibilities and coincidences and straightforward geography.

So in Do! Day 1, we're going to take a fresh look at what we do, why we do it, and how we can work out ways to do more of the things we love, while still paying the bills!

5:2 INSPIRATIONS

HOW MUCH TIME WE SPEND WORKING IN A LIFETIME

As always, it depends which study you read, but statisticians estimate we'll work between 69,000 and 100,000 hours over an average of 40 years in a paid job or career (a lot of the variation is down to gender). Globally, our hours do vary. Here are the average hours worked per year:

Australia 1,693 hours
Ireland 1,543 hours
Japan 1,728 hours
New Zealand 1,762 hours
United Kingdom 1,625 hours
United States – the winners (or losers in leisure time) 1,787 hours

A life's work

What do we do with all that time? A 2013 study by a UK healthcare company found that across their working life, the average worker will:

- take six different jobs at six different firms
- have ten job interviews
- 12 pay rises
- one office romance
- three major arguments with management...
- and 875 small disagreements
- experience three periods of stress

- take 125 sick days including one period signed off work with stress
- be made redundant once
- be unemployed once
- and be late for work 188 times

And somehow we'll also find time to drink 45,500 cups of tea or coffee during working hours...

Happiest professions and most miserable

So, what kind of work will make you happiest? Obviously, we shouldn't generalise – but I'm going to do it anyway! Research from the University of Chicago lists these as the ten jobs with the highest level of job satisfaction:

1. Clergy
2. Fire-fighters
3. Physical/physiotherapists
4. Authors (Ha! Good news for me!)
5. Special education teachers
6. Teachers
7. Artists
8. Psychologists
9. Financial services workers
10. Operating engineers (crane/machine operator)

Another UK study found work in scientific research, health care and technology, or working with children or in the great outdoors offered high levels of job satisfaction! But there's more to it than the industry you work in – your place in the hierarchy and your feelings of control (or lack of it!) play a big part too.

5:2 MYTH-BUSTING

STATUS AND STRESS

I talked about good stress in the Relax chapter (see page 182), but workplace stress can be damaging if we feel we have no control over it.

We might imagine that pin-striped city boys shouting 'Buy! Sell!', or heart surgeons making tiny incisions under bright lights, experience the most pressure. Yet it's not the higher paid, higher-status professions which suffer most from stress-related health issues.

There's a famous study among British civil servants (government employees), called the Whitehall Study. In fact, there were two studies, one starting in the 1960s, and one in the 1980s which is still ongoing.

Both showed that men in the lower paid and lower status grades of job (like messengers, doorkeepers) had higher death rates from all causes, and particularly from cardiovascular diseases, than men in the higher managerial grades. Even when the first study accounted for certain other risk factors which were more likely to be found in the lower grade employees (like obesity, smoking, less spare time and high blood pressure), those employees were still twice as likely to die due to heart disease as their higher status colleagues.

One theory to explain this could be that the lack of control and status in a job may lead to increased levels of cortisol, one of the 'fight or flight' hormones we described in the Relax chapter. Prolonged, raised levels of this could affect the immune system, leaving the cardiovascular system more vulnerable to disease.

As with so many disease risk factors, we don't yet understand the causes fully but it does indicate how critical employment is to both our physical and mental health. So it's logical that unemployment can also have an impact.

Losing your job – losing your identity too?

Redundancy or losing our job is something most of us will experience at some point. And it can be devastating – not just because of the financial consequences but also the effect it has on our confidence and health.

Studies in Finland, the US, UK and Sweden show a range of health problems, and a higher death rate, in those who have been unemployed. The effect was both cumulative – it rose the longer someone had been unemployed – and long term, with effects continuing even after someone found work.

Obviously, the financial side of unemployment is a huge factor. But where people facing unemployment are given advice on how to use the extra time to focus on health, leisure and maintaining the motivation to find work again, it can reduce the negative effects. Exercise can also reduce stress, as can something as simple as living near and appreciating parkland or green space.

It's not easy to stay motivated when you've had the choice about whether or not you can work taken out of your hands. And even *voluntary* redundancy can be a difficult adjustment.

Losing my job – and finding my vocation

I've been through redundancy twice. Both times there was the option to apply for other jobs to avoid leaving, but despite my fears, I sensed that the right, if scary, choice was to make a fresh start.

I'd worked for the BBC for most of my career – and I did secretly feel proud of the fact that people were instantly interested in my job when I mentioned those three famous initials. So after I left, it affected not only my financial security, but also my sense of identity. So much so, that I decided to go back as a freelance the following year. I admit it. I was a bit lost without my old employer!

At the time, the break between jobs felt unproductive. Yet five years later, I realised that my period without work had sown the seeds for my first novel. And when I left my job again, when half my department was also made redundant, I started my second career, as a full-time writer.

Before I was made redundant, there was no way I ever wanted to be self-employed. The idea *terrified* me.

And now? I cannot imagine going back to being an employee.

Self-control – and self-employment

I'm not alone in going it alone – in the UK, for example, the number of self-employed people is at an all-time high, with 14% of the working population freelancing. The economic crisis has been a factor – 367,000 more people were self-employed in 2012 compared with 2008.

It's not always by choice: companies often use freelance-style contracts to get round employment law. And we're not all setting up multi-million pound internet innovations from our bedrooms – in fact, the most common freelance occupations are taxi drivers, farmers and construction workers.

But the 'free' aspect of freelance work can offer many benefits, including choosing your own hours and feeling much more self-reliant. The downsides: those hours are often much longer, and your income is no longer guaranteed…

Working from home, working in the home and retirement

Working *from* home as a freelancer can be fantastic, especially if you have caring responsibilities – but watch out for social isolation and even for weight gain once you stop commuting (luckily I know a very effective diet for that…).

Working *in* the home – caring for family members or running a household – brings its own challenges. Whether you call yourself a home organiser, a carer, a house wife or house husband, or a domestic goddess, it can be satisfying *and* frustrating.

Retirement is different again, though the isolation, lack of work contact and stimulus, and loss of status can be similar emotionally to unemployment. Several studies have shown the importance of hobbies in keeping positive – and keeping diseases like dementia at bay. Even the word 'hobbies' is slightly patronising – there's no reason why you shouldn't approach leisure or unpaid activities with all the passion and commitment that you did paid work.

Making what you do meaningful, wherever you do it

The key, for me, is to look for meaning in what you do – it's why I called this section Do! rather than Work, because it's not just about what we're paid for. Work – paid or unpaid – can give us:

- social contact and friendship
- physical activity/movement
- routine
- purpose
- change of environment
- mental stimulation
- status

Which is most important to you? That's what we're going to explore right now.

Key Activity, Do! Day 1
vocation, vocation, vocation

'Location, location, location' is the key to house-buying – so when it comes to finding work or activities you love, 'vocation, vocation, vocation' is what we need to explore.

Vocation literally means 'calling' or 'summons' but now we tend to think of it as an occupation that has real meaning for us. Medical or faith-based professions are often seen as vocations, but we can broaden that out to mean the occupation or occupations – not necessarily paid – that we feel fit our abilities, interests and beliefs like a glove.

This activity helps you look at your own talents and interests to discover the right job or voluntary activity – or, if you already love your work, how you can make it even better!

Step 1

Write down lists for the following – pick at least three to brainstorm. Try not to worry about feeling boastful – if you have a skill, don't waste it!

A   Ten skills or things I'm good at – at work and outside it.
B   Five things (or more) I love in a work environment.
C   Five things (or more) I dislike in a work environment.
D   Five things that give me energy/make me want to leap out of bed.
E   Five things friends or family always ask me to help with or give advice on.
F   Five ways I make a difference or could make a difference.

Step 2

I hope you're feeling proud of your list – you rock! We all have a unique combination of skills and abilities, not to mention a few preferences (and pet hates) of our own.

- Now take two of the lists you made – and brainstorm jobs or activities that could really use your skills or passions. List A is the most obvious source of ideas but try at least one of the others as they're likely to give more interesting responses.
- Be as wild as possible – write everything down!

I've included some examples on the next page.

Five things that give me energy/make me want to leap out of bed

1 Fresh air/outdoors:
    - Roles: Mountaineer, gardener, fisherman/woman, bicycle courier, hot air balloonist, conservation volunteer, charity-walker on Everest, canned oxygen seller

2 Children playing/laughing:
    - Roles: Nursery teacher, clown, laughter yoga specialist, children's TV presenter, joke book author, volunteer at children's hospital, play therapist, toy shop owner

3 Chocolate!
    - Roles: Chocolatier, assistant in chocolate shop, recipe writer, cocoa bean importer, official chocolate taster, cookie baker, researcher on the science of chocolate, hot chocolate maker

4 Having a party to go to/being the hostess with the mostest:
    - Roles: Personal shopper, tour guide, cocktail maker, gossip columnist, party or wedding planner, pub landlady, host for language students or conference delegates, fund-raising hostess

5 Coming home to the dog's wagging welcome after a long day:
    - Roles: Pet groomer, dog walker, animal charity campaigner, puppy breeder, animal behaviourist, dog chaperone on movies, pet sitter/feeder, animal shelter volunteer, puppy walker for working dogs

> **Five things friends or family always ask me to help with or give advice on**
>
> 1 **Property finding/home renovations:**
>   - Roles: Estate agent, property finder, mortgage adviser, interior designer, project manager, property writer/columnist, decluttering specialist, house clearance
>
> 2 **Make-up:**
>   - Roles: Avon lady, bridal make-up artist, beauty blogger, stage make-up specialist, skincare advisor, facialist, making and selling own lotions or range, volunteer offering makeovers to hospital patients
>
> 3 **Dating and relationships**
>   - Roles: Counsellor, matchmaker, agony aunt, singles night organiser, family mediator, TV relationships expert, sex therapist, magistrate
>
> 4 **Latest music to download:**
>   - Roles: DJ, bar manager, musician, music agent and promoter, trendspotter, music reviewer
>
> 5 **Setting up their computers/phones:**
>   - Roles: Technology engineer, electronics store assistant, app developer, digital 'concierge', users' manual writer, trainer or volunteer to help people get online

See what I mean about being wild with your ideas? It's interesting how one idea flows from another.

What if I already *love* my current job?

Brilliant! I love mine, too. But you can still use elements of this activity to find ways to enjoy it even more: think about the ways you could use other skills that might be underused at the moment – perhaps in your leisure time or through volunteering. Developing other interests can be great for building resilience if you ever go through tricky times at work.

What if I'm retired/can't commit to paid work or there are no jobs in my area?

My example above includes plenty of volunteering ideas – or ways to get more experience to use in job-hunting, or to give you back any of the positive aspects of work that you miss.

Step 3

Simply let those ideas brew while you read the next section. Do add to the lists if new ideas occur to you.

Key Activity

feedback – and how to design your own job

That activity might have thrown up a diverse range of occupations. But where on earth are you going to find a vacancy requiring your own special set of skills?

Maybe the answer is to design your own...

You might have heard the phrase 'portfolio career'. It's a slightly irritating label, but the idea of building a job description made up of different elements and income sources, is exciting.

It's more than possible to make a living or make a difference by combining roles.

There have always been certain jobs and activities where traditional employment is not an option – writing books is one, along with other jobs where you're only as good as your last piece of work – actors, artists and musicians are in the same boat, though the compensation of doing something you love may be enough to keep you going through the lean times.

The joy of inventing your own job description is that you can combine financially risky roles with the ones you already earn from. Here are a few examples of people I know:

- Most of my novelist friends also do something that is a more reliable source of income, like teaching/lecturing in English or writing, mentoring, reviewing, journalism or dog-walking.
- I know… a builder who makes amazing recycled sculptures to sell via the web and local stores.
- A graphic designer in training as a family counsellor.
- A garden landscaper who moonlights as a musician.

Try finding *those* jobs in the situations vacant columns! It won't happen – so, instead you need to…

Write your own job description

The internet has made it so much easier to sell your skills, and even invent whole new job categories. One of my brainstorm examples above was for a role as a digital concierge – basically, helping people with their phones, networks, music and entertainment systems. The idea of that job even ten years ago would have seemed crazy – but now, I'd certainly consider paying someone to help me sort out my wires (which are permanently crossed)!

If you're crafty or creative, eBay and the maker's selling site, Etsy, provide a market for second-hand and hand crafted goods that can showcase your flair. And sites like peopleperhour.com, elance.com and odesk.com offer work in web development, copy-writing and other skills – or you can also search for a freelancer to work on your own project.

Don't rule out combining paid and unpaid work – by applying to be a trustee, a volunteer, a magistrate or local elected representative.

The well-known 'don't give up the day job' advice is very sensible – a hobby can turn into a dream job, but it might not be as much fun if you have to pay the mortgage this way. Trying before you 'buy the life' is a good way to make career decisions that you won't regret.

I wrote novels alongside my day job for three years before I felt confident enough professionally and financially to make the switch, and that removed a lot of the pressure I'd have felt if I'd done it the minute I got a book contract.

In today's challenge, we're going to turn the ideas from the key activity, into actions. Because it's all about doing!

Challenge, Do! Day 1
you are what you do

5:2 is all about small changes, big dreams. Yet job change is a huge change – so it's important to take it step-by-step. For our challenge today, we're going to work out how.

There are three options for you to choose from, depending on your situation:

A is about new career options

B is about growing in your existing job

C is about using your free time in the most satisfying way.

Option A Work out what you're worth!

1 Choose either a job or a service that inspires you from the list you came up with from the Key Activity.

2 Research the demand and potential income:

- If it's a service, is there a site where you can check rates of pay or upload a test advert to see if you get any responses and confirm the level of demand in your area?

- If the work that interests you involves creating or selling a product, research websites or local stores where you could test market your products or makes, and discover the optimal pricing?

- Look for online and face-to-face networks of people doing similar work or producing similar products. Even in competitive worlds, people can be very helpful and are often flattered to be asked (see the bonus activity, Find a Role Model, which is on page 243).

3 Now break down your next steps – list three actions to take in the next week (See 5:2 Inspirations: the power of the pomodoro for more examples on page 53 of how to make big change easier) – and schedule a time to do them.

Option B Make the most of your current job

So, you're one of the lucky worker bees who gets a buzz from their job… but tiny changes can make things even better! Some of these suggestions might seem obvious or trivial, yet we often get so used to our working environment that taking a fresh look can offer simple, effective improvements that make day-to-day life hassle-free.

1 Look at the lists you made earlier, especially: five things I love in a work environment and five things I dislike in a work environment.

2 Consider whether you can find one way to increase the elements you love and one way reduce one of the things you dislike.

   • For example... you love the social element of work, but your current workplace has people from a wide geographical area so nights out are hard. Could you set up a carpool or taxi-share for one night a month or vary where you go out locally so everyone gets a night out close to them every few months?

   • Or you really like your colleagues but the noises in the open-plan office interfere with your concentration when you have a complex report to write. Solution: ear plugs or personal stereo when you need to shut out all distractions!

3 Now think about the skills and talents you use outside work. The best way to become indispensable at work is to extend your skills and keep learning. So, look to your hobbies – whether it's your great new social networking ideas, or your lemon meringue pie, finding a new way to stand out at work will benefit you and your employer.

4 Make plans to implement one of these ideas – the elements you love, hate, or are great at – within the next week.

Option C Find your dream non-job!

Maybe you're not working right now – but you'd love to find all the positive experiences of work… without the long hours or the pressure.

1 Look at the list of ideas from the key activity and then pick two to investigate more thoroughly. Consider the following:

- What opportunities are there locally? If you need to travel, what expenses might be paid?
- What commitment would you need to give – and does it fit in with what you can give right now in terms of time and lifestyle?
- If future employment is an issue, are there training or CV benefits from giving your time for free?
- Or might you use the experience to set up your own business in future?
- Alternatively, will you enjoy what you're doing as an end in itself?

2 Choose the most appealing possibility, and make contact by email or phone right now!

Challenge: feedback

It's tempting to think that when it comes to the big things in our lives – work, relationships, where we live – we need to make dramatic gestures. If you're itching to make a change, then perhaps my cautious approach is disappointing?

Yet you'd be surprised what effect simply sowing the seeds of change can have, longer term. I hope *5:2 Your Life* has helped show that little changes can also have dramatic effects – without the risk or disruption of grand decisions. It's certainly what happened to me…

I love my (second) career as a writer, but it's nerve-wracking at times. The market for fiction has changed a lot lately, and I always love trying new things. A few years ago I did a version of today's key activity. I looked at what interests me outside fiction – and food/cooking and health/psychology came out as the top two. Food and cooking because I love them, health and psychology because my own issues with depression have made me fascinated by how people tick and what influences our mood.

At the time, I really couldn't see how I could use those passions, as I'm neither a chef nor a professional psychologist. But I wonder if, deep down, the possibility of developing non-fiction ideas around food and health had lodged in my brain. When I began to follow an intermittent fasting diet, but couldn't find a book about it, perhaps the memory of that previous brainstorm came back to me – and the result is three books, including this one…

If you haven't had a light-bulb moment yet, be patient. The effects of 5:2ing your life may well inspire you in unexpected ways…

Finally for today, here's a bonus activity based on finding ways to learn from people you admire.

Bonus Activity, Do! Day 1
find a role model

This activity is about being inspired by other people's successes or talents – by finding yourself a role model, or mentor, who can spur you on to achieving what you want in life.

Mentoring is popular in schools to help students see the possibilities ahead, and give them advice and guidance on their future. But why let younger people have all the fun? We can all learn from figures we admire.

And your role model doesn't even have to be alive! You can choose to look for a 'real life' mentor who will be able to give you advice on a new career direction or skill – or, alternatively, you can pick a famous or historical mentor to inspire you from a distance.

Option A Choosing – and using – a real life mentor

Approaching someone to help you can be nerve-wracking – but imagine if the boot was on the other foot. How would *you* feel if someone contacted you, not to ask for a job, but simply to seek inspiration? They say they'd love the chance to talk to you on the phone or buy you a coffee to get advice and to find out how you achieved what you have in life?

It's flattering, isn't it? OK, some potential mentors might be too busy at the moment, or not able to help, but most of us would respond positively to a polite request. The key to finding the right mentor is to work out what you want from one and then make the best approach.

Step 1: working out what you want from your mentor

Jot down answers to these questions:

- **What?** What kind of help are you looking for – advice on starting or building your business, on something specific like branding or exporting? The mentor may share contacts later but it's best to let a mentoring relationship develop rather than expecting the mobile numbers of CEOs.
- **Who?** Do you want someone in your workplace or industry already, or someone to help you go in a new direction? Would you prefer someone of the same gender, or background? Don't rule out people with a different perspective, or someone younger if you're starting afresh.
- **Where?** Do you want someone geographically close, so you can meet, or would Skype/email/phone be a better use of your time and theirs?
- **When?** How long do you imagine the mentoring relationship might last – three months, six months, a year? A mentor will be able to respond best to a clear request and expectations.
- **How?** How will you find them? Research charities, companies or individuals you admire, and find the person's biography online. Ask friends and family if they know someone suitable, as a personal contact can speed things up.

Now, draw up a list of possible mentors – aim for more than one or two in case your first choices are busy or hard to contact – and plan your approach!

Step 2: making the approach

- Email is often the easiest way to approach first of all – **choose your subject line carefully** as it's the first thing the potential mentor, or their team, will see. Try to find something personal that makes it look as little like spam as possible. *Mentoring request from Bristol-based female entrepreneur* might leap out if your potential mentee has Bristol links and is known for encouraging women in business, for example.
- **Be business-like and succinct.** Explain why you want a mentor, and be clear about why you've chosen them. Be confident and friendly but not too pushy.
- Do get a friend or friends to read the email, to check if the tone is right, and to **double-check spelling, grammar and punctuation**.
- Cross your fingers. **Press send**! And now send a second one to the next person (though not to two people in the same company at the same time!).
- After a week, send the briefest of **follow-up emails** – again, polite and friendly.
- If you haven't had a response, **try the next two potential mentors** on your list.
- If you're brave, you could **make a phone call** instead of sending that follow-up email, to 'check your original message didn't get caught in spam'.

Step 3: making the most of your mentor

- Respect their time by being punctual, and well prepared with questions. Don't over-run your slot unless they initiate it.
- Take notes!
- Stick to your original request in terms of the commitment you asked for – let them suggest any extra follow-ups.
- After each mentoring session, send a short email to thank them for their time. And once you get to the end of the mentoring relationship, do send a card or perhaps a small thank-you gift.
- Pay it forward – look for mentoring opportunities to offer to others, or do it informally by sharing advice and information via forums or websites.

Option B Choosing – and using – an iconic mentor

Sometimes the people we admire are out of reach – either because they're famous, or because they're no longer alive!

But that shouldn't stop you using them to inspire you… OK, maybe that feels a bit like being a teenager with pictures of your heroes on your wall – but, when you come down to it, was being inspired by an idol such a *bad* thing?

Step 1: choose your iconic mentor
Geography or availability doesn't matter – it's about what they've achieved and how they've done it.

You don't have to admire everything they did or do – you can choose a work–life balance mentor, a style mentor and a business mentor. As many as you like!

Step 2: focus on one mentor at a time...

- Choose the first mentor – borrow or buy biographies, watch movies or documentaries featuring them, read interviews online, focus on what they can teach you through their actions and words about the world you want to enter.
- Choose a key phrase or quote from your idol to inspire you.
- When you've had enough of one mentor – move on to the next!

Do! Day 1: feedback

That's today done – and it's the last of our 5:2 days to focus on a particular topic – I hope it's given you some inspiration.

Next time, we'll be reviewing all the things you've done over the last six weeks, so do have your notes ready as we look back – and then prepare to go forward!

DO! DAY 2: WHATEVER NEXT?

Today is about celebrating what you've done – and planning all the amazing things you're still going to do.

There's no theory or research to read through today. Instead, we're focusing on your personal experiences and achievements while 5:2ing your life – and working out how you can keep up the momentum. So let's get straight down to it…

Key Activity, Do! Day 2
the pat on the back

Step 1: Review

Take a look at the notes, lists and activities you've put in your notebook and on the 5:2 planner. Find any photos you've taken along the way. Use a highlighter pen, if you like, to make it easier to highlight the most interesting comments. If you've done 5:2 with a friend, then get together for this part. It should be fun!

Take a moment to feel proud of the things you've tried, whatever the result!

Step 2: Evaluate

Now take a fresh sheet of paper and answer the following:

- What has surprised you most?
- Which activity or challenge did you enjoy the most?
- Which activity or challenge was most difficult? Were there any you found emotionally hard?
- Which week did you feel made the biggest difference and why?
- Which week was hardest and why?
- Are there activities or themes that felt particularly relevant to your life – and that you'd like to return to?
- How do you feel overall about what you've done and achieved in the last six weeks?

Step 3: Build

Weigh up how you feel about going forward. Decide if there's a theme or activity you'd like to go back to – or whether you want to build on action you're already taking as a result of *5:2 Your Life:* it could be working on your fitness, getting more involved in your community or looking for a job that is the best match for you.

Key Activity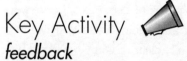
feedback

I really hope you feel fantastic about what you've done.

At the start of the plan we acknowledged that it's normal to feel positive *and* negative emotions when you try different challenges. You might experience that right now, too, as you look back at things that went well and things that could have gone better.

Change can be hard, even when you're choosing to try and make things better. But the rewards, as I hope many of the activities have shown, are absolutely worth it.

A little later, you're going to reward yourself for all your hard work. But before that, there's one last challenge...

Challenge, Do! Day 2
plan to succeed

As you know, I'm a fan of goal-setting (despite never having actually scored a goal in any sport, unless you count air hockey, or the own goal in netball in the Girl Guides).

This final challenge is about setting goals to carry on your good work – now you've completed the programme, you can zone in more specifically on what matters most to you, using the 5:2 tools!

Step 1: choose a priority
Take a look at your ferris wheel/pie from Day 1 and the answers to Step 3 from today's activity and decide what you want to prioritise. It might be immediately clear to you what you'd like to work on next... but, if not, here's a list of possible themes to inspire you:

Movement
Health
Family
Friends
New business ventures

Finance
Creativity
Work volunteering
Work–life balance
Love
Community
Giving back
Fun
Simplifying
Travel
Home comforts

Step 2: brainstorm some aims!

You're an old hand at brainstorming now, so write down some ideas for aims you might set around this priority. Alternatively, there might be activities or challenges you wanted to tackle in the last six weeks but didn't get the chance to try. For example:

- Have dinner with the family twice a week, distraction free.
- Do something scary.
- Try a me-date.
- Do the 5:2 spending diet.

Or you may already have a much bigger goal in mind – to move house, do a charity trek in Latin America, change careers.

In which case, follow the guidance on breaking that down into manageable tasks on page 54.

Step 3: do the SMART thing

Chosen an aim or goal? Now let's make it SMART.

Each letter stands for a way to make your goal clearer:

- **S**pecific – what exactly do you want to do?
- **M**easurable– how will you know whether you've done it?
- **A**chievable – can you do it in the timescale?
- **R**ealistic – is it possible, with the resources and skills you have?
- **T**iming – how long will you give yourself to do it?

For me, measurability and timing are the most important. Here are two examples of what I mean:

- **Have dinner with the family twice a week, distraction free:** that's measurable – let's give it a fortnight – four dinners – and see how it goes!
- **Do something scary:** that's a bit vague, so decide on the exact action that will raise your heart rate in a good way, and commit to trying it by the end of this week.

With longer-term goals, set overall timescales and smaller deadlines:

- Move house: your overall aim might be to achieve this within 12 months, but stay on track with smaller goals:
  - Do outstanding DIY and paint front door – within three weeks.
  - Replant garden and sow seed to patchy lawn – this weekend.
  - Get three estate agent valuations – in one month.
  - Talk to financial advisor about new mortgage – in six weeks.

And so on… carry on with the smaller deadlines and goals until you have the keys to your new front door in your hand!

Step 4: 5:2, 6:1 or every day?

As you've discovered, 5:2 is an easy way to try out small changes, but you can adapt the focus to suit however much, or little, time you have available. Some weeks you might not be able to do much more than re-read your objectives, others you can tick off a task each day. Make a plan now!

Step 5: make it happen!

As a 5:2 Your Lifer, you should be brilliant at achieving your goals by now. But use the motivational tricks we used elsewhere too: sharing your goals with friends, writing them down somewhere you can see them frequently and putting reminders in your diary or electronic calendar will all help!

Bonus Activity, Do! Day 2 celebrate!

You know that bonus activities are normally optional.

This one isn't. Or you'll need a very good excuse not to do it…

Your task is to celebrate what you've achieved. Just as I urged you to take care of yourself by putting together a pleasure list in Week 1 and going on me-dates in Week 2, now I want you to reward yourself for all your efforts. Here are a few ideas:

- **Throw a party for yourself** – invite friends if you want, or have the most indulgent party on your own, playing your cheesiest music and dancing as though no one is watching (because they're not!), eating the party food you love and wearing your favourite frock and a party hat!

- **Create a scrapbook** to celebrate all you've achieved, complete with tickets, pictures and quotes you've found inspiring.
- **Frame a photo** from one of your *5:2 Your Life* activities or challenges, and put it in a show-off place in your home.
- **Buy something nice** that symbolises what you've done – like a charm bracelet, with a charm to represent the different challenges, or new sports gear to wear while you work out.
- **Have a grand day out** somewhere you've always wanted to go!

Not the end, but the end of the beginning...

That's the end of the *5:2 Your Life* six-week plan – well done for completing it. But this isn't the end – it's just the end of the beginning. The positive changes are going to continue.

Don't forget, if you haven't tried the Eating Plan, then that's in Part 3 on page 273 – it's been a life changer for tens of thousands of people, so do take a look.

Part 4: tools for your 5:2 life on page 353 has resources to help you keep 5:2ing, so you could head over there now... or you could enjoy a very well-deserved glass or cup of something nice to drink!

Cheers! And congratulations...

DIY 5:2 YOUR LIFE

What if you know what you want to change – but don't know how?

This section is for you.

5:2 Your Life is designed to be completely flexible – for many people, the structured six-week programme of Discover, Connect, Simplify, Move, Relax and Do! takes them through a process of discovering and tackling their priorities.

But some of us already have a clear idea of what we need to change to be happier – whether it's cutting down or cutting out alcohol or cigarettes, changing career or moving home. We just need more guidance on how to make it happen.

That's where DIY *5:2 Your Life* comes in. You're going freestyle.

Do It Yourself – designing your own programme

In this part of the book, we'll build a focused, personal programme, using the challenges, activities and tools in the main section, but concentrating on your personal aims.

It will mean a bit more planning on your part, as the programme will be unique to you.

The idea is that you can pick and choose the activities you

do, and the sections of the book you read. But don't overlook the benefits of just having a flick through the book, as you never know when something may strike a chord. I'd certainly recommend reading through all the sections over the next few weeks, and making a note if a challenge or technique appeals.

Practicalities

The book would end up *huge* if I repeated all the activities, so you will need to go back and forth a bit to read the relevant parts. You could try using sticky notes to mark the relevant parts.

Start by reading Before you begin: tips and guidelines on page 15 which will explain what you need to *5:2 Your Life*.

Read that? Then you're ready to start.

The first of your DIY *5:2 Your Life* days should be devoted to personalising your programme. It's worth taking the time to do this properly.

My boyfriend often quotes a phrase he uses at work: Proper Planning Prevents (Piss) Poor Performance... you know it makes sense.

DIY *5:2 YOUR LIFE:* DAY 1

To build your DIY programme you need to think about:
- **what** you want to achieve: spelling out what you want
- **why** that matters to you: what your motivation is
- **when** you want to work on it and how long your programme will last
- **who** else you might involve in your plan and who will be affected
- **how** you're going to tackle your aim: the tools and activities you'll use.

Let's look at each of these in turn.

What you want to achieve

You want to put your aim into words. Maybe what you want is simple and easy to define, for example:
- Give up smoking.
- Cut down on alcohol.
- Look for a new job.
- Sort out my debts.
- Move to new area.

Those are clear goals. You'll know when you've achieved them.

But there's a second type of aim that's harder to measure. These tend to be based on changing how you feel. For example, your aim might be:

- have more energy and feel fitter
- feel closer to my partner and kids
- get out of a rut

The first set of aims is easier to plan a programme around. To help you focus on those, you can read about goal-setting in 5:2 and the power of the shopping list on page 34.

You can also use the SMART checklist:

- **S**pecific – what exactly do you want to do?
- **M**easurable – how will you know whether you've done it?
- **A**chievable – can you do it in the timescale?
- **R**ealistic – is it possible, with the resources and skills you have?
- **T**iming – how long will you give yourself to do it?

But what about the second kind of aims, the 'feeling' ones?

One way to help refine your thinking and needs is to try one of the Find your 5:2 focus activities from Discover Week (see page 21). You can also read through and try out some of the options in the Challenge: what's in my way on page 36, which should help you to identify any obstacles to achieving what you want.

Do you now have a clearer idea about the What? Let's go deeper and think about the Why.

Why that matters to you

What we want is not the whole story… *why* we want it is just as important.

An obvious example is money. We might want to have a million pounds in the bank, but for most of us, the money isn't the point (unless you like stroking bank notes!): it's what we can do with it.

So take some time to think through the reasons behind the aims you discovered in the What? section. This will help you to:

- get to the root of what you want, and your aims may change as a result
- imagine the benefits the aim will bring once achieved, which helps motivation.

By asking yourself the questions *Why? What will this give me?* you can increase your chances of success.

In the case of smoking, it may seem obvious.

<u>Why I want to quit smoking:</u>

- Cut my risk of premature death.
- Save money.
- It's a nasty habit.

So far, so good. But the questions will deepen your resolve.

- Cut my risk of premature death.
- *Why? What will this give me?*
- A longer and healthier life.
- *Why? What will this give me?*
- More time in good health to do the things I want in life.
- *Why? What will this give me?*
- More time to see the kids grow up. I want to see my

daughters get married, unlike my father who died before he could give me away. Also time to travel – my aunt was in and out of hospital with health complications for years and couldn't leave her home town. I don't want that.

The *Why? What will this give me?* questions can bring strong emotions and vivid dreams to the surface, and build a stronger motivation to make changes.

Activity: Why? What will this give me?

Take 5 minutes – set an alarm so you take the full amount of time – to ask yourself *why you want to achieve your particular goal.*
- Jot down your answers in your notebook.
- Keep going until you feel like you've got to the root of what you want to achieve: the benefits behind the aim.

Next, it's *When.*

When you want to work on it

How long do you want to devote to your aim?
- Four to six weeks is a good start: the *5:2 Your Life* plan is six weeks long, because it's a doable period of time, but it also gives you the chance to establish new, good habits.

Which days can you work on your aim?
- This is *5:2* so you need to think about two days when you can spend time focusing on your aim – whether that's through activities, by cutting out a habit you want to stop (for example, not drinking on those days) or by seeking out help or support on those days.

Use the 5:2 Planner on page 358 to work out when are the good days for you.

Who else you might involve

Involving others can be very helpful. Read Tell the world or keep a 5:2 secret in the tips and guidelines section on page 15, which explores how to find the right supportive people to involve in your plans.

For your DIY plan, you may want to recruit specialist support around topics like smoking cessation, alcohol issues or conflict in relationships.
- Your family doctor or nurse is the first port of call for anything health related.
- Advice centres like the Citizens' Advice Bureau (CAB) in the UK can advise on debt reduction or legal issues, and put you in contact with experts who won't charge for their services or take a commission.
- Charities dealing with housing issues, alcohol or substance misuse, debt and relationships will be able to offer advice and resources such as books or materials.
- Time-focused campaigns like Stoptober (for smoking) can offer intensive support that makes you feel part of something bigger, which many people find helpful.

- Whatever you're doing, the chances are there's a forum or Facebook group devoted to that common cause. Try joining a few but take it steadily at first, so you can be sure that the tone and objectives of the group are similar to your own, and also that there are no commercial interests dominating.
- Sometimes there's no substitute for the face-to-face support of people with expertise, or those who've successfully tackled similar issues. Your doctor and relevant charities can help you find trustworthy therapists or support groups.

How you're going to tackle your aim

What techniques and activities will you use to help you achieve what you want? There are three areas to take into account.

1 Set yourself activities and challenges

The main *5:2 Your Life* programme works by having one activity and one challenge on each 5:2 day. The activity can involve reading, thinking through an issue and answering questions, or planning something more practical. The challenges are almost always practical and immediate.

It makes sense to plan your 5:2 days in the same way. There are numerous techniques and activities that you can build into your programme as listed on page 264.

Of course, you're free to invent your own challenges or activities that fit your own aims!

2 Challenge and nurture yourself

In the main programme, there's a balance between challenging yourself to do things, and rewarding and nurturing yourself. In Week1, for example, the pleasure list ensures that you schedule in rewards.

Aim to include at least one nurturing/rewarding activity each week.

3 Record and monitor your progress

It is important to record your experiences – including the parts you find hard – and monitor your progress. That also involves trouble-shooting anything you're struggling with.

Here are some tips:

- Use the 5:2 planner to schedule your plans – and use an electronic calendar or your diary as a reminder.
- Then mark up the planner with what you do on each 5:2 day, and any things you're trying out in between.
- Record your feelings and experiences in a notebook.
- Start each 5:2 day session with a short check-in – ask how the week has gone, how you felt about the activities, read through any notes you made last time.
- If you're feeling stuck, try Draw the obstacles (page 36) or Why? What will this give me? (page 259) to tackle any issues that seem to be stopping you doing what you want.

Activities and challenges: the 5:2 Your Life list

Here's a list of the activities, challenges and inspirations in this book.

Read through the suggestions and use your 5:2 planner to schedule the ideas you like. As a rule, activities and challenges involve actions – inspirations can be read at any point to provide… inspiration!

Inspirations, Activities and Challenges:	What it offers:
Inspirations: insights from the end of life (page 25)	A quick reminder of what's important to us.
Activity: find your 5:2 focus (page 26)	An overview of what you want to do during your programme.
Challenge: what's in my way? (page 36)	Different activities to help us understand what's stopping us achieving what we want.
Activity: the pleasure list (page 44)	An exercise to help you work out what you can do to motivate and reward yourself.
Activity: Take 10! (page 50)	An activity to help you blitz through life's irritating tasks.
Inspirations: the power of the pomodoro – or getting organised, one tomato at a time (page 53)	A reading and technique to help us focus on important tasks without getting overwhelmed.
Activity: shrinking the big stuff (page 55)	More on how to break seemingly huge issues into doable chunks.
Inspirations: the Puppy Effect (page 58)	How you can harness the tricks the mind plays to your benefit.
Challenge: The Power of Dreams and Reminders (page 59)	A practical task to help you achieve more.
Inspirations: Who are the happiest people alive? (page 69)	Food for thought on how different factors affect happiness.
Activity: Reaching out (page 72)	Suggestions for making contact and connecting with the people who matter.

Activity: my movement DNA (page 157)	Useful for anyone who wants to be more active as part of their plan.
Activity: move mood board (page 161)	An activity to help you visualise your goals.
Challenge: move! (page 164)	More suggestions for being more active.
Inspirations: habit-forming for beginners (page 170)	Key steps to help you turn bad habits into good ones.
Inspirations: stand up! Sitting down is bad for you (page 168)	A reading on the hidden dangers of staying still.
Activity: get the habit (page 172)	An activity to help you establish new, good habits.
Activity: what can you do for a fiver? (page 177)	An activity to show you can make a difference without a big budget.
Inspirations: what is sleep? (page 185)	The facts about shut-eye.
Inspirations: what mindfulness meditation can do (page 191)	Review of a study of the positive effects of meditation.
Activity: meditation is what you need (page 191)	A really simple but useful exercise you can use to improve well-being and increase levels of calm.
Challenge: Cyber-detox (page 197)	A challenge focusing on electronic distractions (as recommended by 007).
Activity: the big sleep makeover (page 199)	A step-by-step makeover to help you enjoy your zzzz.
Inspirations: rethinking stress (page 206)	An alternative way of looking at how stress affects your body and mind.
Activity: the 5:2 ferris wheel of life (or the 5:2 pie) (page 209)	A visual exercise to see where your life is balanced and where you need more help.

Challenge: get real! (page 214)	Find ways to do more in real life, and less online or alone.
Activity: do something scary! (page 216)	Challenge yourself to do something to get the pulse racing in a good way.
Inspirations: how much time we spend working in a lifetime (page 226)	A great incentive for making the most of your working life.
Activity: vocation, vocation, vocation (page 232)	An activity to help you understand your strengths and passions.
Challenge: you are what you do (page 238)	Practical ideas for improvements, whether you love or hate what you do.
Activity: find a role model (page 243)	Pin-ups aren't just for teens – how to take inspiration from great people.
Activity: the pat on the back (page 248)	Take time to recognise your achievements and feel good about what you've done.
Challenge: plan to succeed (page 250)	Make plans for the next step in your journey.
Activity: celebrate! (page 253)	Mark the end of your plan with a big reward.

Sample DIY *5:2 Your Life* plan

Here is one sample plan, as an example of how you could formulate yours and what you might achieve.

Jim is 46 and has decided to devote four weeks in January to improving his health. But after previous attempts at new year resolutions ending in failure, he's going to try the 5:2 plan this year.

Jim plans out his weeks, but allows a little flexibility to change as he progresses.

Week	Day	Diary/achievements	Activity/challenges
Week 1	5:2 Day 1	Jim reads the Inspirations: insights from the end of life, and the sections on goal-setting and forming good habits. He knows he wants to cut down on his drinking, take some exercise and hopefully improve his sleep over the next four weeks.	Activity: he plans his next four weeks and picks activities he likes. Jim's personal challenge: No drinking on 5:2 days.
	5:2 Day 2	Jim creates a mood board with his kids, pulling in images of a younger Jim looking healthier, plus activities they can do together.	Activity: move mood board. Jim's personal challenge: No drinking on 5:2 days. He's experimenting with new soft drinks to replace the half-bottle of wine he's got into the habit of drinking.
Week 2	5:2 Day 1	Fitness: Jim follows Day 1 of the Move Week — he borrows next door's dog and goes for a country walk.	Normal Move Activities. Jim's personal challenge: No drinking on 5:2 days.
	5:2 Day 2	Fitness: Jim follows Day 2 of Move Week — goes to the local climbing wall with the whole family, and downloads an app that will help remind him to stretch and move while at work.	Normal Move Activities. Jim's personal challenge: No drinking on 5:2 days.

	5:2 Day 1	Relax: Jim reads up on sleep and tries the big sleep makeover, plus a self-guided meditation. He carries the meditation out for 10 minutes and decides to do it again for the next two days.	Activity: the big sleep make-over and meditation. Jim's personal challenge: No drinking on 5:2 days.
Week 3	5:2 Day 2	Jim decides to try expressive writing, which brings to the surface issues around his own father's drinking, but finds after a few days that he feels better, and is clearer on wanting to be healthier and more energetic with his kids.	Tries expressive writing. Jim's personal challenge: No drinking on 5:2 days – goes for a walk instead.
Week 4	5:2 Day 1	Jim uses what he's found out from the expressive writing work to re-prioritise: he writes to his sister, who he hasn't spoken to for several years, and suggests they could meet up again. He also realises he wants to plan a big holiday with the kids while they're still young enough to think he's cool! He tries out the 5:2 spending diet and works out he can save enough for a really good holiday by July.	Writes to his sister. Tries 5:2 spending diet. Researches holidays. Jim's personal challenge: No drinking on 5:2 days.

Week 4	5:2 Day 2	Plan to succeed: Jim has decided to increase the non-drinking days to three per week as he finds them easy to manage. He also decides that for the next four weeks, he's going to be active two days per week, and he books a family introductory scuba-diving course at his local pool and a holiday to Egypt as he's always wanted to dive with the children. Celebrate! Jim buys a smoothie maker with the money he's saved not drinking wine, and holds a wild smoothie party for the family, competing for prizes for most colourful, most delicious and most disgusting.	Signs up for scuba class. Smoothie party! Jim's personal challenge: No drinking on 5:2 days.

PROGRESS:

At the end of the four weeks, Jim has lost 4lb/2kg by cutting out drinking, and saved enough money to book a scuba-diving class.

He's more active at work – walking round his office several times a day has actually made him feel more in touch with his colleagues.

The expressive writing was tough but he's glad he did it as he hopes it's not too late to be closer to his sister.

And he's sleeping better, too… though he hasn't told his colleagues he meditates.

All without signing up to a gym membership or feeling guilty about still enjoying sharing a great bottle of wine with his wife at the weekend.

DIY: over to you

Ready to DIY? If it feels daunting to go it alone, then you can begin by doing the week or weeks that seem most relevant to you, and then pick and choose activities from the other weeks or days that you fancy trying.

Do aim to carry out a 5:2 related activity or challenge on two days a week, to keep the momentum going. And don't forget you can still share ideas on the 5:2 Facebook groups!

Now, if you're interested in the eating plan, turn the page.

3

THE

5:2

EATING PLAN

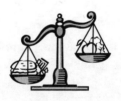

*The proven, flexible approach
to healthy eating that helps
you lose weight and protect
against serious illness,
without guilt or faddy foods*

In this section, you'll find:

- a list of the benefits of the 5:2 Eating Plan
- a quick-start guide
- an Eating Plan checklist
- the 5:2 Eating Plan – daily menus for six weeks of two fast days per week, combining new recipes and simple, everyday meals that complement the themes of each *5:2 Your Life* week
- a section on flexi-fasting, the more flexible way to approach this way of eating.

5:2 benefits: what to expect

Here are some of the positives people experience on the 5:2 Eating Plan

- **Weight loss:** if you have weight to lose, you could drop between 6lb and 14lb (2.5kg to 8kg) during the six-week plan.
- **Appetite control:** becoming aware of your appetite will help you know when you're hungry and when you've had enough.
- **Increased enjoyment of food:** food tastes better and you'll savour it more.
- **Lower food bills:** eating less processed food, and more fresh produce, will cut your bills.
- **Improvements in energy and mood:** many 5:2 dieters have found they have more energy the longer they follow the plan. Our moods can also be more balanced.
- **Reduced symptoms and better health test results:** 5:2

dieters have seen improvements in asthma, menopausal symptoms, thyroid problems – and have seen blood pressure readings and cholesterol test results improve.

- **Potential reduction in risk of serious diseases:** this is a key motivator for many of us – losing weight and fasting both have the potential to cut the risk of chronic conditions including heart disease, cancer, diabetes and dementia. See How does 5:2 affect my health? on page 282 for more information.

Quick-start guide to the 5:2 Eating Plan

What is the 5:2 Eating Plan?

It's the simplest, healthiest, cheapest diet you'll ever try!

5:2 is a flexible approach that cuts your calorie consumption on two days a week – and allows you to eat normally on the other five days.

- **'Fast' days:** These are not total fasts, but a significant reduction in calorie intake, to a limit of around 25% of your normal requirements. You can either calculate your own personal fast-day calorie limit (I explain how on page 282) – or use average energy needs: 500 for women and 600 for men. You can eat this as one, two or three small meals.

- **Normal days:** I sometimes call these 'feast' days because all food feels like a feast after a fast day, but 'normal' or 'non-fast' days are popular with many because it avoids the idea that you pig out the rest of the time!

- **4:3, ADF, 6:1?** You can fine-tune the number of days you fast, depending on how quickly you want to lose weight –

so **4:3** means three fast days, which may increase the speed of weight loss. **Alternate Daily Fasting** is when you fast every other day. And **6:1** is one fast per week, for once you reach your target weight, or if you're doing this mainly for health rather than weight loss.

Why does 5:2 work?

- All weight-loss diets rely on you **consuming less energy** (food, measured in 'kilocalories' – known as calories for short) than you use up in your daily life.
- **5:2 achieves that** – but in a less monotonous way than most full-time diets. **Your life is less restricted** – you can still socialise or cook the foods you love – so you're more likely to stick to it long term.
- It also **reduces the guilt around food** because **no food or food group is banned**, so individual foods are less likely to become an obsession.
- Dieticians estimate that to lose 0.45kg (1lb) of weight, we need to have a 'deficit' of 3,500 calories – and to put the same amount *on*, we'd have to eat 3,500 calories more than we need. If you fast for two days a week, you're aiming to **create a deficit** of just under 3,500 calories each week.
- That deficit may increase on 5:2 as many of us naturally eat less on the other days, once **we're more aware of our appetite and healthy eating**.
- On the other days, you can **eat whatever you like, but not in excessive quantities** – awareness of what you're eating, without guilt, is the best approach to avoid 'cancelling out' the benefits of fast days by eating far too much on other days.

When should I fast?

- **Most of us fast twice a week** – but look at flexi-fasting on page 346 for an alternative approach.
- **Most 5:2 dieters separate their fast days** – for example, doing Monday and Wednesday or Tuesday and Thursday. It's easier to stick to your limit when you know that tomorrow you can eat what you like. Though once you're used to fasting, you can do the two days together.
- **You don't have to do the same days each week**; fit them around work commitments or family occasions.

What and when can I eat on fast days?

In principle, you can eat whatever kinds of food you like – as long as you stay under your calorie limit. However, it makes sense to eat wisely.

What:

- It's best to focus on vegetables and small portions of protein, like lean meats, fish, eggs or tofu, which are more satisfying and keep us fuller for longer.
- Remember, many fruits and refined carbohydrates like white bread or rice are best avoided because they're not as satisfying – and sweets, cakes or alcohol are definitely not fast-day friendly, as they're high in calories and may cause a sugar rush that makes you crave more food.

When:

- You can consume your calorie allowance in one, two or even three meals, although the health benefits may be greater if you restrict yourself to just one or two meals.
- Many 5:2 dieters – me included – have found that it is

easier to postpone eating until lunchtime or later. Others eat at breakfast and dinner. It's your choice.

Will I get hungry?

- Your limit of 500 or 600 calories is enough to keep you satisfied, if you choose wisely.
- But fast days can be strange at first. We're so used to eating at regular times, and snacking or grazing between meals, that many of us have forgotten how it feels to have an appetite. It can be an unsettling feeling but there are a few things to bear in mind.
  - Hunger tends to come in waves and if you have a hot drink or distract yourself with a phone call, a piece of work or a quick look at the online 5:2 groups or forums, it will soon diminish.
  - This is a temporary choice you're making and one from which your body will benefit long term.
  - Getting back in touch with your appetite can help you develop a healthier attitude to food. Allowing yourself to get hungry, and anticipate meals, means food tastes amazing – and you're more aware of when you've had enough, not only on fast days but all week long.
  - Finally, remember the 5:2 catchphrase: *tomorrow you can eat what you like!*

Are there other side effects?

All changes in diet bring about changes in how our body works, which is why **you should check with your doctor that there's no reason not to begin (and see the warning on page 2).** Do check if you have any chronic conditions or a history of eating disorders. I know of people with both Type 1 and Type 2 diabetes who have found ways to fast under supervision but you need to check with your specialist or diabetes nurse. You should not fast if you are pregnant or breastfeeding.

You may find that on the first couple of fast days you experience:

- Headaches: diet headaches are very common with any change in eating patterns. Drinking lots of water can help.

- Digestive changes: some people have found that when they're not eating as much, they don't need to open their bowels as regularly – or that when they break their fast, they need to 'go' soon afterwards. This usually settles down.

- Feeling cold: this is quite common, and may be caused by the fact that digesting food creates heat in the body – so when you're digesting less, you're producing less heat. Hot drinks and soups are the best remedy for this, when the weather is cold too.

- Sleep changes: sometimes, you may struggle to sleep on a fast day – try eating a small snack a couple of hours before bed.

- Short temper: changes in blood sugar and unfamiliar feelings of hunger can make us feel snappy. Build non-food treats into your first few fast days (a magazine to read, a walk round the block), and plan a couple of emergency snacks if you really need them. See the list on page 347 for some ideas.

- If you feel very unwell, don't hesitate to stop fasting until you've seen your doctor but this is very, very unusual.

5:2 Fast-day tips

- **Plan your fast days in advance** – at first, choose days when you're busy but not flat out. Avoid days with social commitments where you might be tempted to eat out or have an alcoholic drink.

- **Plan your fast-day *foods* in advance, too** – the Eating Plan will help!

- **Drink plenty** of water, or black coffee or tea, herb teas and diet drinks. Count the calories in milk, and be aware that some dieters do avoid milk and artificially sweetened diet drinks as they may cause insulin spikes that could increase your appetite.

- **Experiment with the number of meals you eat**. I prefer two or even one single meal as it helps reduce hunger pangs for me, but I couldn't have faced that to begin with.

- **Exercise is possible** on fast days – many of us run or go to the gym, but take it easy at first and stop if you feel unwell. Calories burned during exercise can't be added to your fast-day limit – stick to the normal limit and feel very virtuous!

- Studies suggest that dieters who **keep a record** of what they eat tend to be more successful. You can jot this down in a notebook or use an app or website like MyFitnessPal.com: simply enter the name of the food or scan the package barcode, and the app calculates the total number of calories (though as most of the calorie counts are provided by users, some entries may be unreliable).

- MyFitnessPal also allows you to **record your weight and measurements over time**. However, it doesn't have a setting for 5:2, so it may tell you to eat more on a fast day. The easiest way to overcome this is to set your membership to Maintain, and ignore the warnings on fast days!

Calculating your personal energy needs

Many people get good results on fast days by sticking to the average limits of 500 calories for women and 600 calories for men. That figure is based on consuming around one quarter of what an 'average' body needs in calorie terms per day. But you can easily calculate your own figure, which is known as Total Daily Energy Expenditure (TDEE).

- Being taller, shorter, heavier or more/less active than average will affect how many calories you need. A smaller woman who does no exercise will need significantly fewer calories than a taller, overweight woman who is training for a marathon.

- **The easiest way to do this is using an online calculator** to work out your energy expenditure (TDEE). See Part 4: Tools for your 5:2 life or the 5:2dietbook.com website.

- You then divide that total by 4, and that's your calorie limit for your fast days. Though it is a guideline – if you exceed it by fewer than 50 calories/10%, you should still lose weight.

- Using this calculator will also help you understand **how much you can eat on a non-fast/normal day without undoing your hard work on a fast day**. I don't recommend calorie-counting every day – but knowing your TDEE helps give you a guideline.

- Different online calculators may give different results because there are two different formulas, but the variations aren't huge.

- If you lose a lot of weight, you should recalculate your limits, as your TDEE decreases along with your weight – *unless* you step up your activity levels, which may happen as you find you have more energy and confidence!

How will 5:2 affect my health?

Weight loss is the most obvious result of 5:2, but that doesn't mean it's the most important. Your fast days will also have a startling effect on your body's ability to repair itself.

- Research from human and animal studies has shown that intermittent calorie restriction (the general term for 5:2-style regimes) can reduce the risk of developing many cancers, cardiovascular diseases and Alzheimer's disease and other forms of dementia.

- Fasting triggers processes which slow down the growth of new cells, and instead boost repairs to our existing ones, to prime us for survival.

- Our ancestors' lives followed a feast/fast pattern, so our bodies adapted to take in as much energy as possible in the good times, like after a successful hunt or harvest. By feasting, our bodies would accumulate fat stores in reserve to keep us going during the leaner times.

- Now we have a wide choice of foods and in many countries, famine is non-existent – yet we're programmed to crave sweet, fatty, high-energy foods.

- 5:2 reintroduces those 'rainy' days – and it appears that our bodies respond by trying to ensure we're in the best shape for famine. That includes 'tidying up' rogue cells that are cluttering up the place, and repairing any that need help.

- In addition, leaving gaps between eating may help. For years, many diet gurus have encouraged us to snack between meals, to maintain blood sugar. However, this means the body is constantly having to use insulin to balance our blood sugar levels. Insulin prevents levels of sugar becoming dangerously high – but it also stops us burning fat. Fasting means our bodies have less work to do, and when insulin isn't circulating, we can start burning our fat stores for energy.

- Intermittent fasting also improves insulin sensitivity. This is good because we want our bodies to be as sensitive to insulin as possible, so we respond faster and more efficiently. It's one of the key factors in reducing our risk of developing Type 2 diabetes.
- Research suggests that fasting may also protect against dementia, including Alzheimer's.
- 5:2 may also increase mental sharpness and energy – and even have a positive effect on the chemicals and processes that play a part in depression and other mood disorders.

You can read much more about these processes in my book, The 5:2 Diet Book.

What weight loss can I expect?

It depends on how long you follow 5:2 for, and your weight to begin with. There are several ways to assess whether your weight could be damaging to your health.

- Body Mass Index (BMI) is the one most commonly used by doctors: the chart in resources will show you your measurement and whether that indicates you are overweight or obese.
- BMI is not perfect, however, and another indicator is your waist measurement. 'Pear-shaped' people, with larger hips and thighs, may have lower risks of heart disease/diabetes than 'apples', who store more fat around their belly and may also have more visceral fat around the vital organs. One simple guideline is that we keep our waist measurement to less than half of our height, or a ratio of less than 0.5.

You measure at the point midway between the bottom of your ribcage and your hip bones. For example, I am 163cm (64in) tall, so my waist measurement should stay under 81.5cm (32in).

It's hard to face the scales or use a tape measure when you feel bad about your weight, but once you begin to lose weight, you'll be glad that you were honest with yourself because your progress will be all the more impressive.

Our forum members vary in speed of weight loss – some lose 2.25kg (5lb) or more in their first week, and others never lose more than 0.2kg (0.5lb) a week. I lost slowly, at a rate of less than 0.5kg (1lb) a week on average, but am now 2 stone lighter than when I started. In general, people with more weight to lose are likely to see more rapid losses, while that last little bit before your target is often the toughest to shift.

The other five days: guidance on what to eat, and how much

On 5:2, you're advised to eat normally on the other five days, and your diet can include your favourite foods... but what does 'normal' mean? Should you calorie count? And what can you eat on your five days?

The simple answer is: you can eat your favourite foods and you don't have to calorie count. I still enjoy chocolate, cheese, treats, celebratory meals and wine, though I've found removing the guilt and any restrictions has made my eating much, much more balanced overall. I don't binge on my feast days; everything I eat feels like a feast and I savour my food, but I stop when I'm full.

The more complicated answer is: it can be easy to cancel out the calorie deficit you've created on your fast days if you eat an awful lot on your normal/feast days. For us to become overweight in the first place, our normal diets must have included too much of the wrong things. Here are a few guidelines:

- 5:2 can't change how our body uses up energy: if you eat more calories than you're burning off, you will gain weight.

- For many of us, fast days help us develop more awareness of how much food our body actually needs and when we're full.

- But some of us have spent so many years (or decades) on calorie-counting diets that we're nervous about having no restriction.

- If you do want to count on normal/feast days, then your TDEE (Total Daily Energy Expenditure) is roughly what your limit will be. The averages are 2,000 for women and 2,400 for men, but if you're shorter or smaller than average, or less active, it may be quite a bit lower. Mine now I've lost weight is round 1,700 calories. Calculate this (see Calculating your personal energy needs on page 282), then add up your calories on a couple of days – perhaps a week day and a weekend day, and see whether your calorie count seems about right. However, don't get too hung up on exact numbers: remember your intake will vary naturally day by day depending on your activity levels, social commitments and so on.

- Be carb-aware – all foods are not the same: some have far more nutrients than others. I now tend to eat fewer of the refined carbohydrates, including bread, rice, pasta and desserts, because I know they may make me hungry again pretty quickly. But if I want them, I enjoy them. That freedom means I can imagine doing 5:2 for life, unlike low-carbohydrate plans which create guilt around certain foods.

- When it comes to treats like wine, chocolate, cake or other high-sugar foods, ask yourself whether you're eating them because you want them, or simply out of habit or because they're there. If you do want some, try to slow down the eating so you enjoy the taste – and see if you can get the same enjoyment from a slightly smaller portion than you'd have served before.

Try to move towards the freedom of trusting your appetite and instincts longer term.

What if my weight loss stalls?

- Remember that your weight may fluctuate on a daily basis for many reasons.
- Our bodies vary day-to-day depending on what we've been eating, and for women, hormonal changes can add 2.5kg (5.5lb) or more at different times of the month! Many of the happiest 5:2 dieters on our forums only weigh themselves once a month, or not at all, instead relying on their tape measure, the fit of their clothes and compliments from friends and family to help them monitor their progress!
- If you go for three weeks without weight loss (and you are still definitely overweight), try adding up the calories you're eating on an average normal/feast day. If it's a lot over your TDEE (or the average of 2,000 for women and 2,400 for men, which is based on someone of average height, weight and activity levels who may also be fairly active), then try to identify small ways to cut back on normal/feast day consumption without feeling you're missing out.

Certain medical conditions can make it harder to shift weight, so if you are confident you are following the plan correctly, it's worth discussing it with your GP.

How long can I stay on 5:2?

For as long as you like. For me, and many others, it's simply our routine now, not a 'diet'. Once you reach a healthy weight, you might like to shift from 5:2 to 6:1, i.e. just one fast day a week.

Where can I get more support?

For specific medical issues or questions, be sure to consult your doctor, nurse or specialist.

For general support, the 5:2 Facebook groups are brilliant – I've never come across such a generous, well-informed bunch. We'd love you to join us! Find the Facebook group at www.facebook.com/groups/the52diet – it's free to join.

The 5:2 Eating Plan checklist

5 THINGS 2 DO BEFORE YOU START

1. **Have you talked to your doctor or practice nurse**, especially if you are on medication/have an ongoing condition?

2. **Have you chosen two days in the next week for your fast days** – use your diary to find days that are busy but not excessively so, without any big social occasions. Mark the days in your diary or use the 5:2 planner.

3. **Have you planned your meals for that day?** Do the shopping in advance and plan a couple of emergency snacks or drinks in case you need them, from the extra rations section on page 343.

4. **Have you recorded your weight and measurements** so you can monitor your progress? And do you have either a notebook or an app ready to record your fast-day eating?

5. **Are you focused, with a support system in place?** Think about telling a friend or supportive family member who can remind you why you want this. Or join an online forum or Facebook group. It can also be a great idea to try Find Your Focus activities (pages 26 to 35) from the

5:2 Your Life plan so you're focused on what you want to achieve...

Done all of that? Then it's ready, steady, 5:2!

The 5:2 Eating Plan in action: tips and guidelines

Each week, there are menus for two fast days.

They have been designed to complement the work on the *5:2 Your Life* plan, so the dishes are energising in Week 4, for example, to support the focus on being more active!

But remember, you can design your own menu if you prefer. Flexibility is the name of the game with 5:2 – see 5:2 Flexi-fasting – doing it your way on page 348 to help you plan your own version.

The recipes are a mix of fish, chicken and vegetarian options. Eggs and fish are used often as they're a great source of protein, without being too high in fat or calories. Fruit also features, but mainly berries as they give a delicious burst of sweetness without too much sugar!

Most days add up to 500 calories – on occasion they are a little under or over, but as you learn how many calories are in foods, you can experiment yourself! And men can add an extra 100 calories per fast day – see page 345 for guidance on this.

Oils and fats

Fats push up the calorie counts on fast days, yet they're important in cooking (and in your diet generally). I use a 1-calorie spray, an emulsion of fat and water. You can buy these in supermarkets. You spray onto a cold pan – they look white, because of the emulsion – and then heat and cook as normal, though it's best to avoid very high temperatures. Alternatively, you can get a pump spray and fill it with olive oil, but this will be higher in calories.

I haven't included 1-cal spray in the calorie counts for the recipes because how much you use depends on the size of the pan.

When I want a little additional flavour, I will use 'real' fats and count the calories. Olive oil is good for dressing and roasting, while coconut oil, which is solid at room temperature, is easy to spoon into a pan and adds a subtle flavour to spicy dishes. It may also have positive effects on diabetes and brain function, and have anti-microbial properties.

On measurements and calorie counting

On your fast days, weighing your food is important and informative, especially at first. I have a small digital scale and weigh everything in grams, so I can get very accurate measurements.

Sometimes the quantities I've listed look extreme – 3g of nuts or seeds, for example – yet it's amazing how much difference a few pine nuts or a little cheese can make. Awareness is the key: it's important to be informed about what each food offers us in energy terms – and energy is what calories measure. Oh, and one small point: what most of us call calories are actually *kilo*calories, which is why nutrition labels use the abbreviation 'kcal'; packaging sometimes gives figures in Kilojoules or kJ as well, so double-check.

However careful you are with your measurements, you can never be 100% certain how many calories you're consuming. The same ingredients from different companies can vary, so the counts will always be approximate.

In all recipes where there are alternative ingredients, we've used the lowest calorie options to provide the calorie total for the dish.

All dishes serve 1 unless otherwise stated.

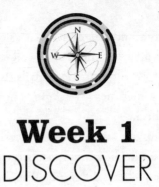

Week 1
DISCOVER

On the menu...

This week, the two fast-day menus offer three small meals for each day... with a focus on discovering great flavours to ensure you are getting the most taste for your calories.

Don't forget, men are allowed a precious 100 more calories than women. Either choose an extra ration from page 346, or simply be a little more generous with portion size or extras like nuts, seeds or cheese.

To drink: you can choose water, diet drinks (try to avoid too many of these), black tea or coffee, herb teas (most are under 5 cals) but count calories in any milk you use – I like almond milk as a great lower calorie substitute.

Fast day 1

Breakfast
Berry 'smoochie' with oats and raspberries (120 cals)

This is halfway between a smoothie and a porridge pot: like a big comforting smooch. Soak the oats overnight to make them digestible (just pop them in the glass you're going to serve it in, to save washing up!).

> 15g oats, 53 cals
> 50g almond milk, skimmed milk or apple juice, 7–18 cals
> 50g raspberries (or any berries), frozen or fresh, 20–30 cals
> ¼ banana, around 30g, 32 cals
> 1 tablespoon fat-free Greek yogurt, 8 cals

Pour the milk or juice over the oats the night before and leave in the fridge (you can prepare enough for two mornings and simply use half).

In the morning, add the other ingredients and whizz up in a jug blender or using a hand blender. Drink and go!

Lunch:
Harissa roasted veg with sweet-mint yogurt cooler (129 cals)

This is absolutely yummy and so filling, especially on a cold day. Harissa is a spicy chilli paste that can add flavour to meat, fish and, as here, vegetables. Roasting the veg makes the most of their flavours, and the cooling sauce with metabolism-stabilising cinnamon is a great counterpoint to the heat of the harissa. I like rose harissa best.

Vegetables for roasting: for example, ½ red pepper, ½ yellow
    pepper (30 cals), 1 small courgette (20 cals), 100g
    mushrooms (13 cals), ½ red onion (19 cals)
1-cal spray
1 teaspoon harissa paste, 20 cals
2 tablespoons fat-free Greek yogurt, 20 cals
Handful chopped mint leaves, 5 cals
¼ teaspoon ground cinnamon, 2 cals

Serves 1 but double up and you can eat this tomorrow with a melted goat's
cheese topping and crusty bread, or serve to the family as a side dish tonight.

Preheat oven to 200°C/400°F/gas mark 6.

Quarter the peppers and remove the seeds and stalks. Then cut all the veg into
even sized chunks (the mushrooms can stay whole if they're small).

Spray a baking sheet with 1-cal spray, then mix the veg in a bowl with the
harissa paste. Arrange the coated veg on the sheet. Bake for 40 minutes, using a
spatula to turn the veg over once halfway through cooking time.

For the cooler, mix the yogurt in a small bowl with the mint leaves and cinnamon. Serve on the side or drizzled over the veg.

*Extra ration: a mini wholemeal pitta bread (80 cals) goes well with this, so you
don't waste any of the spicy sauce.*

Dinner

Sticky sesame salmon or tofu with citrus green beans (230 cals)

This delicious nutty and sweet dressing works perfectly with
salmon, and adds flavour to tofu if you prefer a veggie dish
(it'll be lower in calories, but check the packet for the exact
count). For a hotter, citrus flavour, replace the soy sauce with

lime juice, and add half a teaspoon of crushed chillis to the marinade.

½ teaspoon sesame oil, 22 cals

½ teaspoon honey, 10 cals

1 tablespoon soy sauce (5 cals) or lime juice

½ teaspoon dried chilli flakes (optional)

1 fresh or frozen salmon fillet (100g), 140 cals, or 120g tofu,
    100–150 cals

1-cal spray

Veg:

100g fine green beans, 27 cals

Grated rind and juice of ½ a lime, 10 cals

½ teaspoon sesame seeds, 16 cals

Mix together the oil, honey, soy sauce and chilli flakes (if you're using them). Defrost the salmon fillet, if frozen, or slice the tofu into strips. Drizzle the sesame sauce over the fish or tofu and leave to marinate in the fridge – overnight is best.

Spray 1-cal spray onto a non-stick frying pan, then heat to a medium temperature. Cook the salmon or tofu for 8 minutes, or until cooked through. Turn the salmon to make sure it doesn't burn; with the tofu, you can let it brown at the edges, to give more texture.

Meanwhile, boil a small pan of water and trim the beans. Cook or steam the veg till tender but still crunchy (4–5 minutes) – drain, then toss in the juice and rind. Serve with the fish/tofu, with sesame seeds sprinkled over the top.

Tip: double up on the marinade – it keeps for several days in the fridge and can be used on chicken or other fish too.

Fast day 2

Breakfast
Poached egg on 1 slice wholemeal toast with Marmite (138 cals)

Simple but yummy, a well-poached egg is a thing of beauty. If you hate Marmite, you could add a few baby spinach leaves instead.

   1 small slice wholemeal bread, 55 cals (25g slice from smaller loaf)
   1 medium egg, 78 cals
   Splash of vinegar (not malt)
   Scraping of Marmite, 5 cals (leave out if you hate it)
   Salt and black pepper

Toast the bread. Poach the egg: bring a medium saucepan of water to the boil over a medium heat. Add a splash of vinegar. Break your egg into a small bowl or cup. Create a whirlpool in the water with a fork or whisk and, with your other hand, slip the egg into the middle of the pan as gently as possible. Turn down the heat and set a timer for 3 minutes. Check the white is set before removing the egg from the pan, and set on some kitchen paper to absorb the excess water.

Spread a sparing amount of Marmite (or place some baby spinach leaves) on the toast, top with the egg, salt and pepper.

Lunch

Great big green salad with beans, crispy ham and herb dressing (125 cals)

A simple but generously portioned salad given va-va-voom with crispy ham or spicy beans, and a dressing that tastes far richer than the calories suggest.

> 1 slice Parma ham, 31 cals, 1-cal spray and 30g mixed tinned beans, 34 cals
> OR
> 60g–100g mixed tinned beans, 67-110cals
> 1 large sliced spring onion, 5 cals
> Small handful chopped herbs, e.g. parsley, coriander, tarragon, 5 cals
> Salt and black pepper
> Squirt of lemon juice
> 70g bag green salad leaves, 15–20 cals
> ½ cucumber, sliced or cut into batons, 15 cals
> 25g raw mange tout or sugar snap peas, 10 cals
> 2 teaspoons creamy herb dressing (see below), 10 cals

For ham: Preheat the grill to medium. Lightly oil a baking sheet with 1-cal spray. Place the Parma ham on the baking sheet and grill for 3–4 minutes, until crisp. Remove and set aside to cool.

For beans: Empty beans into a colander and wash thoroughly under running water. Tip into a small bowl (reserve the rest to use later, or marinade the whole lot and use later too) and add the spring onion, chopped herbs and plenty of salt and black pepper plus a squirt of lemon juice.

Toss together beans, salad leaves and vegetables. Crumble the grilled ham over, if using, then drizzle the dressing on top.

Creamy herb dressing (5 cals per teaspoon)

> 50g light cream cheese (e.g. Philadelphia Light with Garlic and
>   Herbs), 73 cals
> 1–2 tablespoons finely chopped fresh herbs, 5–10 cals
> 2 tablespoons semi-skimmed milk, 14 cals
> juice of ½ lemon, 7 cals

Whisk ingredients together in a bowl, or easier still, put them in a jam jar, replace the lid and shake well! Will keep for at least four days in the fridge with the lid on.

Dinner
Tandoori chicken/tofu with cauliflower rice (197 cals)

> 30g/2 tablespoons tandoori paste, 35 cals
> 30g/2 tablespoons fat-free Greek yogurt, 16 cals
> 100g small chicken breast, 120 cals
> OR
> 120g tofu/chicken-style Quorn fillet, 90–120 cals
> 1 whole tomato or 4 cherry tomatoes, 16 cals
> Chopped coriander and 1 dessertspoon fat-free yogurt to serve,
>   10 cals

Mix the paste and yogurt together in a small bowl, then add the chicken/tofu, coating both sides with the mix. Marinate in the fridge for at least an hour, preferably overnight.

Heat the oven to 200°C/400°F/gas mark 6.

To bake, place the chicken breast/tofu onto a sheet of aluminium foil, spooning all the marinade around it. Chop the tomato, or halve the cherry tomatoes, and place these around the chicken/tofu. Crumple the edges of the foil so it creates a little 'bowl' to collect all the cooking juices. Bake for 20 minutes, checking the chicken is cooked through. The marinade will now be quite watery, from the yogurt and tomatoes, so before serving, tip the marinade into a small bowl or mug and, using a fork, mash together. Spoon the marinade over the chicken/tofu, garnish with coriander leaves and yogurt, and serve with cauliflower rice.

Cauliflower rice (16 cals per serving)

This is a brilliant substitute for 'real' rice – I was sceptical but there's very little, if any, cauli flavour. You can whizz the whole cauli in one go, store it in a plastic box and use the other portions within 24 hours.

Serves 2
½ head small cauliflower (approx. 130g), cut into florets, *32 cals*

Grate or finely chop the cauliflower florets until they resemble rice grains. (The fastest way to do this is using the chopping blade or grater in a food processor, but it will result in a finer texture that's a little more like couscous. Pulse to make sure it's not over-processed.)

Cook on full power in microwave for 2 minutes in a lightly covered microwavable dish (reduce to 60 seconds if preparing one portion). Don't add water: there's already enough water in the cauliflower to stop it drying out.

If you don't have a microwave, steam the cauliflower pieces in a steamer (with fine holes, so the grains won't fall through) for 2 minutes, or, stir-fry in a hot pan – with a splash of water to prevent it from sticking – for 2–3 minutes, until softened.

What to expect this week

- Weight loss of between 1lb and 5lb.
- To be very aware of what you're eating – and to experience some hunger pangs at times.

- A great sense of achievement when you complete your first fast day!
- You may get headaches or feel the cold a little more – drinking plenty of lower-calorie fluids, including hot drinks in colder weather, will help reduce that.

Week 2
CONNECT

On the menu...

This week's *5:2 Your Life* theme is connecting with the people and the world around you – reaching out. So I've planned the menus around comforting foods that make you feel good and can easily be shared – the chicken dish and the pizza are both great for family meals, so there's no need to feel left out when you're fasting!

Many of us also find that eating two meals, plus perhaps one snack, works best on Fast Days, so this week you can try that, to see if it works for you.

Fast day 1

Brunch
Balancing cinnamon porridge with cherries (147 cals)

Cinnamon is one of those scents that make you feel warm inside – it smells of home cooking (there's even research showing it could turn men on!). There's also some evidence it can help with diabetes control by balancing blood sugar, and has anti-viral and possible cancer-fighting properties.

Combined with cherries and a little almond, there's more than a hint of Bakewell tart in this breakfast dish! Like the other porridges, it may be easier to prepare in larger amounts and keep portions covered in the fridge for two to three days.

25g porridge or jumbo oats per serving, 90 cals
¼ teaspoon ground cinnamon, 2 cals
75g skimmed milk, 28 cals
OR
75g almond milk, 10 cals
OR
75g apple juice for the cold version, 28 cals
50g cherries (frozen can work with this too), stoned, 30 cals
½ teaspoon almond essence, negligible cals
2.5g of ground or flaked, toasted almonds, 15 cals

Prepare the porridge cold or hot, as you prefer.

Hot version: Cook the oats with the milk and ground cinnamon in a small pan: bring to the boil, then simmer for 3–5 minutes. Stir in the cherries, almond essence and ground almond once cooked.

Cold version: Soak the oats with the cinnamon in the juice or almond milk overnight in a small bowl in the fridge.

Next morning, add the cherries and stir in the almond essence and ground almonds.

Dinner

Golden paprika chicken or Quorn with sweet pepper and spring onions (301 cals)

This is a colourful, tasty dish, full of Spanish flavour thanks to the smoked paprika (the kind that comes in the red tins!). The butternut squash makes a low-cal alternative to potatoes; you can use frozen, but it will go a little mushier, so you add it later during the cooking process, at the same time as the stock. It's good for non-fasting family members too, served with rice.

1-cal spray

½ onion, chopped, 19 cals

1 clove garlic, crushed, 4 cals

140g chicken breast pieces or 2 Quorn fillets, 168/90 cals

1 red or yellow pepper, core and seeds removed, cut into strips, 30 cals

100g butternut squash, cut into small cubes, 40 cals

½ teaspoon smoked paprika, 2 cals

½ teaspoon Dijon mustard, 3 cals

½ teaspoon tomato puree, 2 cals

10ml sherry or wine vinegar, 1 cal

100ml chicken or vegetable stock (e.g. made with ½ teaspoon Marigold bouillon powder), 6 cals

1 tablespoon ½ fat crème fraîche (26 cals) plus a few snipped parsley leaves to serve

Spray a medium non-stick saucepan with 1-cal spray. Fry the onion and garlic for 2 minutes over a medium heat, stirring to make sure they don't burn. Add the chicken, peppers, squash and paprika to the pan and cook for 4 minutes.

Add all other ingredients except the garnish and turn up the heat till the liquid boils and the sauce reduces to half the quantity. Then turn down to a simmer, cover the pan, and cook for 15–20 minutes, checking occasionally to make sure the chicken isn't sticking (if it is, add a little more water or stock).

Check the chicken is cooked through, then serve topped with the crème fraîche and herbs. Cauliflower rice is a good addition to this.

Plus: 1 snack from the Emergencies and craving busters list on page 345.

Fast day 2

Brunch
Avocado and tomato tartare (132 cals)
or with smoked salmon (187 cals)

I wanted to find a savoury breakfast that didn't rely on eggs – and this fits the bill. A tartare is usually uncooked chopped meat or fish, but this is a veggie version though you can add smoked salmon too. Avocado sometimes gets a bad press because it's high in fat for a vegetable, but that means it staves off hunger pangs. This is simple but delicious, a little like a garlic-free guacamole. It's best in late summer when tomatoes are at their tastiest.

> 1 'baby' avocado (or half a small one), around 99 cals
> A few fresh parsley or basil leaves
> 1 ripe tomato or 4 sweet cherry tomatoes, 16 cals
> ¼ of a cucumber, 7 cals
> Sea salt
> Fresh ground black pepper
> Juice of ½ lime, 10 cals
> OR
> 1 tablespoon soy sauce, 6 cals
> Optional: 25g smoked salmon, 55 cals

Chop the avocado, herbs, tomatoes and cucumber as finely as possible, keeping each item separate on the chopping board. Chop the salmon too, if using. Allow excess water to drain away from the tomatoes and cucumber. Sprinkle or grind a little salt or pepper on top of all the vegetables, and the salmon if using, then squeeze the juice or soy sauce onto the veg, making sure the avocado is well coated (to reduce browning).

Find a small ring cutter (the kind you use for cutting out small biscuits – if you don't have one, simply line up the ingredients on the plate). Plate the cutter on a plate, spoon the chopped tomato inside as one layer, then the herbs, then the cucumber, then the avocado and finally the salmon, if using.

Cover with cling film and chill in the fridge for at least 1 hour. Then lift the cutter off and serve.

Tip: if you use soy sauce, then try adding a little pink pickled ginger (the kind used with sushi) to the avocado or salmon mix.

Lunch/afternoon

1 snack from the Emergencies and craving busters list on page 345

Dinner

Square pizza with garlic mushrooms, pine nuts and truffle oil (302 cals)

These 'Wizza' pizzas are one of the most talked about topics on the 5:2 Facebook page – they use a particular brand of flatbread, made by UK brand Warburton's, as a substitute for a pizza base. Then the toppings are up to you. If you don't live in the UK, flour or corn wraps work as well, though be careful as thinner bases may burn sooner.

They're also popular with all the family as you can get the kids involved in choosing their own toppings!

My version here omits the usual tomato flavouring, and uses mushrooms, mozzarella and garlic. There are two more unusual ingredients – pine nuts, which have a delicious, resinous flavour, and truffle oil, which intensifies the mushroom taste so well. But it's delicious without – use olive oil instead.

100g mixed mushrooms, e.g. field, chestnut, button and shiitake, 13–25 cals

1-cal spray

1 clove garlic, crushed, 4 cals

1 Warburton's square wrap, white or brown, 159/187 cals (or other tortilla)

40g half-fat mozzarella cheese, 64 cals

5g pine nuts, 35 cals

1 small handful fresh parsley or chives (or a mix), snipped with scissors, 5 cals

½ teaspoon truffle oil or olive oil, 22 cals

Black pepper

Optional: serve with salad: 25g rocket, 6 cals

1 tablespoon balsamic vinegar, 5 cals

Preheat the oven to 200°C/400°F/gas mark 6. Preheat a baking tray in the oven for 5 minutes.

Chop the mushrooms into equal sized chunks – spray a medium non-stick frying pan with 1-cal spray, then add the mushrooms – cook over a medium heat, turning the mushrooms only occasionally so they brown at the edges.

When they begin to release liquid, after 3–4 minutes, remove from heat, add the crushed garlic (don't add it before this point as it could burn) and return to a much lower heat to cook for 2 minutes till the liquid evaporates.

Place the wrap on the baking tray. Slice the mozzarella as thinly as possible and lay half on the base of the wrap. Top with the cooked mushrooms, add the remaining cheese, and then bake for 7–9 minutes. Dry fry the pine nuts in the frying pan, taking care they brown but don't burn.

Remove the pizza from the oven, sprinkle over the nuts, herbs and the truffle oil. Season with black pepper. Serve with the rocket, and balsamic vinegar as a dressing.

Alterative toppings (use MyFitnessPal or packaging to work out the calories)

Base layer and cheeses:

Tomato puree
Pesto
Lower fat cream cheeses
Reduced fat cheddar or very thin shavings of parmesan-style cheese
Crumbled feta cheese or goat's cheese

Veg and meat:

Roast veg including peppers, onions, carrots and courgettes: use the same method as with harissa veg on page 296, drain away liquid before adding to pizza
Cooked chicken or ham, cut into small chunks or slices
Pepperoni/veggie pepperoni or sausage
Tuna (with sweetcorn or red onion)

Flavouring/toppings to add after cooking:

Dried herbs and spices, including chilli flakes, oregano, marjoram, chives and Italian seasoning
Jalapeno peppers from a jar, sliced, or chilli sauce

Fresh leaves, e.g. baby spinach leaves, rocket
Tinned, drained slice of pineapple or tablespoon of sweetcorn

What to expect this week

- Weight loss of between 1lb and 5lb.
- Fast days will probably feel slightly easier now you have completed two...
- ... but if you're struggling, join a forum or Facebook group for support and on the spot ideas! Completely in tune with our desire to connect more and feel part of different communities.
- And don't forget that the Connect activities in the 5:2 Your Life Plan are a great distraction from any hunger pangs!

Week 3
SIMPLIFY

On the menu...

The *5:2 Your Life* plan looks at simplifying your life – and your finances – this week, so the meals are focusing on best value... great dishes that balance cost and taste. Yet the dishes are still surprisingly exotic, thanks to a mix of seasonal elements and luxurious ingredients preserved in more economical ways. People can be snobbish about freezing or canning but both these methods often preserve food at peak ripeness, and save time and money compared to buying, and sometimes wasting, fresh!

Fast day 1

Breakfast
Chilled harvest porridge pot with hazelnuts (180 cals)

This is a variation on porridge with autumn flavours – choose seasonal fruits for the best value combination. Like the other porridges, it may be easier to prepare in larger amounts and keep portions covered in the fridge for two to three days. You can make a warm version: use milk or almond milk instead of the juice and cook as for Balancing cinnamon porridge on page 304. Use cinnamon, too, if you like it.

25g porridge or jumbo oats, 90 cals

75g apple juice, 28 cals

1 plum, 40 cals, or a small dessert apple, 60–80 cals, depending on size

3g chopped, toasted hazelnuts, 20 cals

¼ teaspoon cinnamon (optional), 2 cals

Soak the oats in the apple juice overnight in a small bowl in the fridge.

Next morning, grate the apple (sprinkle the other half with a little lemon juice to stop it browning) or chop the plum into small pieces. Top with the hazelnuts.

Lunch

Heart-warmer carrot soup with fennel and two gingers (57 cals per serving)

Make a pot of this and freeze the other portions – **this makes 4 servings**. If you don't have fennel, celery is fine. Doubling up on the ginger (fresh and dried) gives a lovely flavour but if you only have dried or fresh, that's fine. Taste as you go and add a little or as much as you want depending on how much you like the heat of the ginger!

1-cal spray

1 onion, chopped, 38 cals

Thumbnail sized knob of ginger, peeled and grated, 4 cals

4 large carrots (around 400g), peeled and chopped into 1cm rounds, 136 cals

Half a fennel bulb, around 75g, thinly sliced (set aside the fronds), 23 cals

OR

1 stick celery, 8 cals
½ teaspoon ground ginger, 2 cals
900ml hot vegetable stock (e.g. made with 2 teaspoons
    Marigold bouillon powder), 24 cals

Spray a large non-stick saucepan with 1-cal spray. Heat to a medium temperature and add the onion and fresh ginger. Fry gently for 1 minute, then add carrot, fennel and ground ginger and fry gently for another 3 minutes.

Add the hot stock and bring to the boil. Simmer for 15–20 minutes or until the carrot pieces are tender. Then liquidise in a jug blender, or in the pan using a hand blender. Top with the fennel fronds to serve.

Dinner

Veggie sausages with mash and mushroom sauce (260 cals)

This is a comforting dish for a chilly day, that won't derail a fast. The mash is a really tasty alternative to potatoes, with a nutty, slightly aniseed flavour, and the sauce is an intensely flavoured alternative to traditional gravy: it's less thick, but the mushrooms are very tasty. Porcini mushrooms can be expensive, but buying smaller pieces is much cheaper. And they keep for ages.

Veggie sausages have really improved in flavour over the years – I like Quorn ones which are tasty and lower in calories than meat versions – but as they don't usually contain much fat, I recommend frying them in a little olive oil or using 1-cal spray, to help them crisp and caramelise nicely.

I've given quantities for two, because it's fiddly to make gravy and mash for one, but you can reheat the gravy and mash in the microwave if you want to eat two single meals. Always cook the sausages from scratch, though.

Serves 2

Sausages (141 cals per portion)

1-cal spray
OR
½ teaspoon olive or coconut oil, 45 cals
2 veggie sausages per person, 140 cals (check label, calorie counts vary)

Mash (98 cals per portion)

1 large carrot, around 100g, peeled and chopped, 34 cals
½ celeriac, peeled and chopped (around 300g), 42 cals per 100g, 126 cals
1 tablespoon hot creamed horseradish sauce, 35 cals
Salt and pepper

Onion and mushroom sauce (21 cals per portion)

150ml hot vegetarian stock (e.g. made with ½ teaspoon Marigold bouillon powder), 6 cals
3g Porcini mushroom pieces (optional), 10 cals
1-cal spray
½ onion, finely chopped, 19 cals
A few sprigs fresh thyme/sprinkling of dried (or oregano/ rosemary)
25g mushrooms, finely chopped, 4 cals
¼ teaspoon Marmite/yeast extract (optional), 3 cals
Pepper

For the sauce, make the stock in a jug or bowl, using hot water, and add the porcini pieces, if using. Leave to soak for at least 10 minutes.

Spray a small non-stick frying pan with 1-cal spray and cook the sausages over a medium heat, according to the instructions. Let them brown but not burn.

Boil the carrot and celeriac in a large pan of water till tender (around 15 minutes). Drain, then mash in a bowl with the horseradish, salt and pepper. To get a fine puree, you can blend in a food processor, with a little of the cooking water.

Spray a small non-stick pan with 1-cal spray and fry the onion and mushrooms over a low heat for 3–4 minutes. Add the stock, herbs and chopped mushroom, plus Marmite if using, to the pan. Increase the heat and let it simmer for a minute or two until the Marmite has dissolved and the sauce is a little more concentrated. You can blend with a hand blender for a smoother sauce (you may need to add a little more water), or serve as it is. Season with pepper, but if you've used stock and Marmite, it won't need salt.

Serve with the sauce on the side or poured over the sausages and mash.

Fast day 2

Breakfast
Tangy mango and cranberry smoothie with almonds (104 cals)

Fresh mangos are expensive, though cheaper from shops specialising in Asian or African produce. Frozen mango, however, is very affordable and keeps the costs and preparation time right down. If your blender can handle ice, this turns into a breakfast 'frozen' margarita so you could even serve it in a cocktail glass. Lighter versions of cranberry juice contain less sugar so a rebound is less likely, and a little ground almond adds texture and more nutritional content.

> 100g fresh or frozen mango (allow to defrost overnight if your
>   blender isn't strong enough to blend ice), 60 cals
> 150ml light cranberry juice, 12 cals
> 5g ground almonds, 32 cals

Whizz the ingredients together in a jug blender or in a beaker with a hand blender.

You can add a handful of blueberries (20 cals) or a quarter of a banana (around 30g, 35 cals) to vary the recipe, though the banana version is sweeter.

Lunch
Ras el hanout baked squash with feta and pomegranate (185 cals)

Ras el hanout is a spice blend from North Africa – it means 'head of the shop' and should be the most aromatic spices the seller in the souk has to offer. You can try this recipe with paprika or curry powder instead, but I love this combination: it's sweet, spicy, salty, crunchy and soft… a real mini-feast if you like pumpkin or squash (I do; the boyfriend loathes it). The colours alone make the dish so uplifting – but squash can be a pain to prepare. I cheat by using frozen chunks, though the edges will caramelise more with fresh.

200g butternut squash, fresh or frozen, 80 cals
½ teaspoon olive oil, 22 cals
½ teaspoon ras el hanout spice mix, 3 cals
25g reduced fat feta cheese, 45 cals
5g pumpkin seeds, 29 cals
½ teaspoon pomegranate molasses, 6 cals
OR
1 tablespoon fresh pomegranate seeds, 12 cals
Fresh herbs to garnish

Heat oven to 200°C/400°F/gas mark 6.

Cut the squash into cubes approximately 3cm square.

Mix the olive oil and spice mix in a small bowl. Add the cubes and coat with the oil – it won't be even because we're being sparing with the oil, but that doesn't matter.

Bake for 30 minutes, until the squash is tender. Turn once during the cooking time.

Turn onto a plate and crumble the feta on top, then the pumpkin seeds. Dot the molasses into the squash and top with a few snips of fresh herbs – mint or parsley work well.

Dinner

Cupboard-love curry with chickpea, mushroom and spinach (198 cals per serving)

Frozen vegetables, and tinned pulses, are cheap and nutritious – and you can turn them into tasty, spicy meals in the blink of an eye! Add good value mushrooms and you have a warming, filling veggie dish. This makes two portions – keep one, covered, in the fridge for up to two days and reheat in the pan or microwave till piping hot.

This dish can also convert mushroom-haters. One of our testers served it to her teenaged son, who has loathed mushrooms for as long as she can remember. The browning technique made them less mushy – and he's asked for this again!

Serves 2

1-cal spray

OR

½ tablespoon coconut or olive oil, 22 cals

100g button or chestnut mushrooms, 13 cals

1 onion, chopped, 38 cals

2 garlic cloves, chopped, 8 cals

3cm/1¼in piece ginger, grated, 2 cals

1 tablespoon tomato puree, 5 cals

½ teaspoon each of ground coriander, ground cumin; 1 teaspoon turmeric, 7 cals

50ml reduced fat coconut milk, 36 cals (counts vary so do
    check your tin)
1 small (215g) tin chickpeas, drained, 164 cals
200g spinach (frozen or fresh), 50 cals
Juice of 1 lemon, 19 cals
5g sesame seeds, 32 cals

Spray a medium non-stick pan with 1-cal spray, or use coconut oil, and heat to a medium temperature. Add the mushrooms to the pan and cook for 3–4 minutes, stirring less than you'd expect, so the edges of the mushrooms are browned. Reduce the heat: add the onion, garlic, ginger, tomato puree and spices and cook for 4 minutes. As you're using a small amount of oil, watch the garlic and spice so it doesn't burn.

Add the coconut milk and chickpeas, and frozen spinach if using. Cook for 4 minutes, till the spinach is defrosted and the chickpeas hot. Otherwise cook for 3 minutes, and add fresh spinach and cook for 1 further minute.

Stir through the lemon juice, then serve topped with the sesame seeds.

What to expect this week

- Weight loss of between 1lb and 3lb (though this varies so much from person to person): sometimes in the third week, any rapid weight loss from the first two weeks may begin to stabilise which is normal with any change in eating.
- Any unwanted symptoms from fast days are likely to be reduced or eliminated by now and the extra energy from fasting will start to kick in, as you begin to enjoy the feeling of control!

Week 4
MOVE

On the menu...

This week, the *5:2 Your Life* plan is focused on getting you moving... so in the Eating Plan we're suggesting dishes that energise and keep you satisfied for as long as possible!

Men, don't forget your extra ration from the list on page 346, or a slightly larger portion (e.g. you could double up on berries and oats in the first recipe).

Fast day 1

Breakfast
Awesome oatsome berry pot (135)

Oats and berries are good choices for fast days when you need to be active, as they are lower GI (Glycaemic Index) foods, which means you should stay fuller for longer. The seeds help, too – be sparing as they're high calorie but pumpkin and sunflower seeds are also nutritious.

This is quite fiddly made in smaller quantities so you can make 2 or 3 portions in advance – have 1 portion on a fast day, and 2 portions on the next normal day!

25g quick cook porridge oats, 90 cals

75g almond milk, 10 cals

OR

75g skimmed milk, 28 cals

OR

75g apple juice for the cold version only, 28 cals

50g berries (frozen is fine – but place in fridge overnight to
   defrost), 20–30 cals

Optional: 1 tablespoon fat-free Greek yogurt per serving,
   8–10 cals

A scattering of seeds or chopped nuts, approx.
   ½ teaspoon/2.5g, 15 cals

Hot version:

Cook the oats with the milk in a small pan: bring to the boil, then simmer for 3–5 minutes. Stir in the berries, top with the yogurt, if using, and seeds or nuts.

Cold version:

Soak the oats in the juice or almond milk overnight in a small bowl in the fridge.

Next morning, add a layer of berries, a layer of yogurt and top with the seeds or nuts.

Lunch

Broccoli and cream cheese velvet soup with chilli pumpkin seed swirl (53 cals per bowl, plus 29 cals for seeds = 82 cals)

I love the contrast of the creamy soup against the spice of chilli sauce and the crunch of the pumpkin seeds.

This makes 4 bowlfuls – it's easier and more practical to make soup in larger quantities, and you can freeze the soup or keep, covered, in the fridge for two days. On a normal/feast day, add a little grated cheese to the top and serve with crusty bread! Reheat gently to avoid the cheese separating.

Serves 4
1-cal spray
1 onion, chopped, 38 cals
1 head broccoli with the toughest part of stalk removed, broken or cut into small florets (around 280–300g), 90 cals
A little grated nutmeg
900ml hot vegetable stock (e.g. made with 1 teaspoon Marigold bouillon powder), 12 cals
50g light cream cheese, 72 cals
To serve: hot Jamaican-style chilli sauce to taste, 5g pumpkin seeds per bowl, 29 cals

Spray a medium non-stick saucepan with 1-cal spray and cook the onion on a medium heat for 2 minutes, then add the broccoli. Grate a little nutmeg into the pan, and cook the vegetables for a further 2 minutes before adding the hot stock.

Simmer, covered, for around 15 minutes until the broccoli is soft.

Use a hand blender to blend the soup together. Lower the heat and stir in the cream cheese till melted.

Pour into a bowl: add chilli sauce to taste and a scattering of pumpkin seeds.

Dinner

Fajitas unwrapped with chicken or Quorn (228 cals per serving + accompaniments)

I love sizzling fajitas in my local Mexican restaurant – and if you take away the flour tortillas, and make some clever substitutions, you can get the taste, with far fewer of the calories. It makes most sense to cook double quantities here and share it – a non-fasting dinner guest could even enjoy a tortilla wrap or two, if you let them! Or this will keep overnight and can be reheated in the microwave or oven, making sure the chicken or tofu are piping hot.

For speed, it makes sense to use shop-bought salsa for this dish – the fresh ones are tasty, and the ones in jars can also be surprisingly fresh-tasting! Though for a salsa recipe, see my *Ultimate 5:2 Recipe Book.*

Serves 2

200g chicken breast, 240 cals

OR

4 plain Quorn fillets, 180 cals

½ teaspoon each of: smoked paprika, ground cumin, hot chilli powder or flakes, 5 cals

Juice of a lime, 20 cals

1 teaspoon olive oil, 45 cals

1 red pepper, 30 cals

  1 yellow pepper, 30 cals

  100g mushrooms (button or chestnut are fine), 13 cals

1 red onion or a small bunch of spring onions, trimmed, 38 cals

1 medium courgette, cut in half width-wise then sliced into strips, 34 cals

1-cal spray

Sea salt and freshly ground black pepper

Serve with all/any of the following:

2 tablespoons of salsa, fresh or from a jar, 10–20 cals

2 tablespoons of reduced fat crème fraîche, 52 cals

1 baby avocado, sliced, around 99 cals

Cut the chicken breast or Quorn into strips. Mix the spices with the lime juice and olive oil. Add the chicken/Quorn strips and coat, and leave in the fridge to marinate overnight or for at least half an hour.

Core the peppers and cut into strips; cut the mushrooms in halves or quarters (unless they're very small) and slice the onion into thin wedges.

When you're ready to cook, spray a large non-stick pan with 1-cal spray, heat to high, and add the veg. Let them sear for 2–3 minutes, only moving them when they begin to smoke and they brown at the edges.

Now add the marinated chicken or Quorn, making sure any extra marinade is tipped into the pan. Cook over a high heat for a further 6–8 minutes, till the chicken is cooked through. If the food begins to stick, add a little more lime juice, or a splash of water.

Season with salt and pepper. Serve with the salsa, crème fraîche, and thin slices of avocado.

Fast day 2

Breakfast
Brunch-time baked egg with basil and sun-dried tomato (138 cals)

This is quick, easy and tasty – set it baking while you hop in the shower. As an extra ration, a mini pitta bread toasted in the toaster and then cut into strips makes 'soldiers' to dip in the egg!

8g sundried tomatoes (vacuum packed, not the kind in oil), 13 cals
A few leaves of fresh basil
1-cal spray
1 egg, 78 cals
1 tablespoon half-fat crème fraîche, 26 cals
Salt and pepper
5g finely grated Parmesan cheese, 21 cals

Snip the sun-dried tomatoes into small pieces, and tear the basil leaves into pieces too. Preheat the oven to 180°C/350°F/gas mark 4. Spray the sides of a small ramekin with 1-cal spray.

Place the tomatoes and basil leaves in the base of the ramekin. Carefully crack in the egg, spoon the crème fraîche on top, season well and scatter with the Parmesan.

Bake for 12–15 minutes, until the white has set but the yolk is still runny. Serve immediately.

Microwave method:

Prepare as above, but make sure you carefully pierce the egg yolk with the prong of a fork or a toothpick (otherwise it will explode!). Cover with a lid or some kitchen paper and cook on high for 30 seconds.

Check the egg and then cook for a further 20 seconds. The white should be set and the yolk still runny. If not, give it another 10 seconds. Don't be tempted to microwave in a 1-minute burst, as it will cook too quickly. An overcooked egg is the fastest way to ruin your fast day!

Lunch

Hot, sour, spiced roast aubergines with juicy tomatoes (111 cals per serving)

This makes a tangy, light lunch dish. To make it go further, serve with bread or rice, or add chickpeas or green lentils from a tin at the same stage as the tomatoes for more protein. If you're making the roast veg on Day 1, then roast the aubergine on a separate tray at the same time, remove the skin, mash, then set aside, covered, in the fridge for up to two days before the final stage.

If you don't have all the spices, experiment with what you have!

Serves 2

1 medium aubergine, 110 cals (cal count is for flesh only)

200g ripe tomatoes (you can skin these if you prefer a smoother
    texture) or 1 small tin, 40 cals

1-cal spray

OR

½ teaspoon coconut or olive oil, 45 cals

2 cloves garlic, crushed, 8 cals

Small piece of grated ginger (around 1cm), 5 cals

Scant ½ teaspoon each of: garam masala, black mustard seed,
    ground coriander, whole cumin, chilli flakes, 10 cals

1 red onion, thinly sliced, 38 cals

Juice of ½ lime, 10 cals

Salt and pepper

A few coriander leaves to garnish

Add half a drained 400g tin of cooked green lentils (113 cals)
    or serve with a mini wholemeal pitta (80 cals) or a portion
    of cauliflower rice (16 cals) to make a bigger meal

Roast the aubergine on a baking tray until soft – around 20–25 minutes at
200°C/400°C/gas mark 6.

Transfer to a bowl and let it cool then peel away the skin. Mash with a fork till
it's fairly smooth.

Chop the tomatoes. Spray the 1-cal or heat the coconut oil in a medium non-stick
pan to a medium temperature and add the garlic, ginger and spices. Cook for 1
minute, then add the sliced onion and cook for 2 more minutes. As you're using
a small amount of oil, watch the garlic and spice so they don't burn.

Now add the aubergine puree and cook until the spices and veg are well mixed.
Add the tomatoes and pulses if using, and cook for 7 minutes. Stir in the juice,
season with salt and pepper, garnish and serve.

Puy lentil salad with beetroot and chilli goat's cheese
(271 cals per serving)

Earthy and delicious! The quickest way to make this is using tinned or pouch-cooked lentils so the measurements are given for 2 servings.

Serves 2

½ 250g pack vacuum packed cooked beetroot (not the kind in vinegar), 50 cals

2 tablespoons balsamic vinegar, 10–20 cals

40g mild soft goat's cheese, 108 cals

1 teaspoon chilli flakes, 5 cals

250g pouch of cooked Puy lentils, 325cals

30g rocket, 7 cals

1 red onion, finely chopped, 38 cals

Salt and pepper

Cut the beetroot into edible wedges and place in a serving bowl with the balsamic vinegar, leave to marinate (you can do this overnight in the fridge).

Cut the goat's cheese into thin rounds and sprinkle with the chilli flakes. Chill.

When ready to serve, cook the lentils over a low heat until just warmed through. Tip on top of the beetroot in the bowl, add the rocket and chopped onion and mix through. Season.

Top with the goat's cheese and serve: if serving over two meals, you can keep the ingredients separate till ready to eat, or the beetroot will 'bleed' – it won't do any harm but doesn't look as pretty.

What to expect this week

- Weight loss of between 1lb and 3lb, though don't be disheartened if you don't lose every week…
- … it's very likely you'll be feeling the difference now in your clothes, and may even be getting compliments about how well you look, or people saying you've lost weight!
- Remember that what's happening *inside* the body can be as exciting as external signs. Many people report reductions in blood pressure readings and fewer symptoms of chronic conditions.
- If you're following the Movement part of the plan on page 168, then being more active should boost your self-esteem. But remember you can't 'earn' more calories with exercise on a fast day – stick to the limit and feel very proud of yourself!
- Around now, your fast days will begin to feel like part of your routine – perhaps you can imagine carrying these on after the six-week plan is complete (I certainly did… now 22 months and counting!).

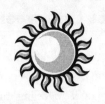

Week 5
RELAX

On the menu...

In the *5:2 Your Life* plan, we're looking at reducing unnecessary stress, and improving our sleep. So I've designed this week's menus around foods that may support the body and aid better rest. Over the years, many claims have been made for foods with miracle healing properties, and I am naturally sceptical, but luckily all the ingredients in this week's plan are delicious too, so there's no hardship in trying them out!

Fast day 1

Brunch

Peppered portobello mushrooms with poached egg (145 cals)

A simple but tasty brunch dish with lots of flavour: eggs help support the nervous system, and mushrooms boost immunity, which can be weakened by stress.

> ½ teaspoon olive oil (you can use 1-cal spray but olive oil adds flavour), 22 cals
> 1 clove garlic, crushed, 4 cals

1 teaspoon Worcestershire sauce, 5 cals
A few whole peppercorns, lightly crushed
2 portobello/field mushrooms, 36 cals
Splash of vinegar (not malt)
1 egg, 78 cals
Salt and black pepper

Heat the oil in a small non-stick pan and fry the garlic over a medium heat for 2 minutes. Lower the heat, then add the Worcestershire sauce and the peppercorns and mix together, then add the mushrooms, stalk side down and cook for 4 minutes. Turn the mushroom over and cook for 3–4 minutes on the other side. If the pan gets a little dry, add a splash of water.

Meanwhile, bring a medium saucepan of water to the boil over a medium heat. Add a splash of vinegar. Break your egg into a small bowl or cup. Create a whirlpool in the water with a fork or whisk and, with your other hand, slip the egg into the middle of the pan as gently as possible. Turn down the heat and set a timer for 3 minutes. Check the white is set before removing from the pan, and set on some kitchen paper to absorb the excess water.

Top the mushrooms with the egg, season then serve.

Dinner

Turkey and Parma ham melt with lemon and olive broccoli (251 cals)

Turkey may contribute to a decent night's sleep because it contains the amino acid tryptophan, which plays an important role in the production of neurotransmitters, which govern mood and sleep.

Turkey is also a good fast-day choice as it's low in fat. This 'sandwich' mixes ham, cheese, herbs and turkey in a delicious grilled melt and is accompanied by a side dish of fresh broccoli with a lemon and olive topping. The sage is a nod to a dish my dad used to make, a 'sandwich' of ham, sage and veal or chicken slices, adapted from the Italian saltimbocca – which means 'jump in the mouth'

Turkey breast fillet, around 100g, 110 cals
20g half-fat mozzarella, sliced very thinly, 32 cals
A few fresh sage leaves or Italian herb seasoning
1 slice Parma ham, 31 cals
100g broccoli, 32 cals
10g drained, pitted black olives, 15 cals
½ teaspoon olive oil, 22 cals
Zest and juice of ½ a lemon, 9 cals
Sea salt and freshly ground black pepper

Heat the oven to 200°C/400°F/gas mark 6.

Create a 'pocket' for the cheese in the turkey breast by cutting a flap along the length of the meat, leaving it attached at the other edge. Lift, place the sage leaves and cheese slices inside, then close.

Wrap the Parma ham around the whole turkey breast. Place the fillet on a baking sheet and bake for 18–20 minutes. Check the breast is cooked through before serving.

Meanwhile, fill a small saucepan with water and boil or steam the broccoli until tender (around 4–6 minutes depending on how you like it). Slice the olives to form little 'rings'. When the broccoli is cooked, drain it, then add the oil and lemon juice to the hot pan, along with the olives, and toss in the hot oil and lemon for no more than a minute. Season and garnish with the lemon zest to serve.

Supper treat
Cherry berry sleep compote (83 cals)

This is a sweet treat for an hour or two before bedtime. Cherries may improve sleep quality by stimulating the production of melatonin, and combined with spices like cinnamon and vanilla, this is deliciously comforting. This makes two servings – serve the second with porridge or with ice cream or pancakes the day after a fast!

Quark is a soft cheese with a tangy flavour that works well with the cherries – or use reduced-fat fromage frais.

Serves 2
150g cherries (fresh or frozen), stoned, 90 cals
50g blackberries or blueberries, fresh or frozen, 20–28 cals
Finely grated zest and juice of ½ a small orange, 30 cals
1 teaspoon honey, 20 cals
½ teaspoon ground cinnamon, 5 cals
½ teaspoon vanilla or almond essence, 2 cals
To serve:
1 tablespoon/15g quark low-fat soft cheese per serving,
    10 cals (optional)

Place all the ingredients in a small, heavy-based saucepan. Heat gently and allow to cook for 8–10 minutes. Tip into a bowl and allow to cool a little – serve warm or cold, topped with the quark.

Fast day 2

Lunch

Courgette pasta with pesto and tomatoes (111 cals)

I *love* this way of saving calories, upping your veg intake *and* enjoying a rich sauce. Because the courgette here isn't a sauce on the pasta – it's the 'pasta' itself, providing a low-fat and low-cal alternative to wheat pasta, and saving you at least 150 calories that you can then 'spend' on a rich sauce. And you don't get the slump that can come after eating a carb-based meal. Plus courgettes have a soothing quality, and the sprinkling of cheese on top contains B vitamins, which help support the brain and nervous system.

> 1 courgette (170g), 34 cals
> 1 large, ripe tomato, chopped, or 5 cherry tomatoes, 16 cals
> 2 teaspoons/10g fresh or bottled green or red pesto,
>   20–45 cals
> 5g Parmesan cheese, 21 cals
> 1-cal spray
> A scattering of pine nuts (around 10 nuts), 20 cals
> Sea salt and freshly ground pepper

To prepare:

Wash the courgette and cut off the stem and base. The simplest way to do this is to use a normal veg peeler, pressing hard so you end up with thicker slices than you would if you were simply peeling the courgette. It can take a bit of practice… Cut strips running top to bottom, moving the courgette as you slice, to get a nice green strip on each 'noodle'.

An alternative is a special julienne peeler that cuts spaghetti-like strands that taste even yummier – and can be used for salads too. I love mine, and if you like this recipe, it could be worth the cost (under £5), though be careful as they are very sharp!

To cook:

Bring a small pan of salted water to a rolling boil, drop the ribbons into the water and boil for 45 seconds–1 minute, depending on how thinly they're sliced. Drain well, and return to pan to season before serving. Or, you could fry the courgette strips in a non-stick frying pan. Spray the pan with 1-cal spray and heat. Toss the ribbons in the pan and make sure they're spread across the base. Cover the pan with a lid, turn down the heat and let them cook for 1 minute before turning the ribbons over and cooking for a further minute on the other side. (I prefer this method.)

Remove from heat, stir through the tomatoes and pesto sauce, scatter the cheese and pine nuts over the top, season with salt and pepper.

Dinner

Salmon, fennel and pea risotto with pink peppercorns
(357 cals per serving)

Pink peppercorns aren't peppercorns at all, but come from a different type of shrub. Let's not hold it against them – they look lovely and their spicy, fruity flavour is a great match for salmon, and also delicious in salad dressings. Or use fresh black pepper if you don't want to splash out on the pink version.

The omega-3 fatty acids in salmon are beneficial to mental function, and fennel may balance female hormones.

It makes sense to cook this for 2, because it's a bit time-consuming: great for a weekend supper dish. Vegetarians can substitute their favourite vegetables for the salmon – mushrooms, asparagus, baby carrots or young leeks, or simply stir a little fresh pesto through just before serving. Serve with a rocket or watercress salad.

Serves 2
1-cal spray
1 white onion, peeled and finely chopped, 38 cals
50g sliced fennel, 15 cals
OR
1 celery stick, finely chopped, 6 cals
1 garlic clove, finely chopped, 4 cals
150g Arborio rice, 510 cals
30ml white wine, 21 cals
350–400ml hot fresh vegetable stock (e.g. made with
    1 teaspoon Marigold bouillon powder), 12 cals
75g petit pois (frozen is fine), 38 cals
30g smoked salmon (offcuts are fine for this, or chop into small
    pieces), 66 cals
Zest and juice of ½ a lemon, 9 cals
A dozen or so pink peppercorns
Optional: 1 tablespoon light cream cheese, 22 cals (additional
    11 cals per portion)

Spray a little 1-cal spray into a large, heavy-based, non-stick saucepan. Fry the onion and fennel/celery for 2–3 minutes over a medium heat, until softened but not coloured. Turn down the heat, add the garlic and fry for another minute.

Add the rice and stir for 2 minutes. Turn up the heat, pour in the wine and heat for a couple of minutes.

Then begin adding the hot stock, a ladleful at a time, waiting until each one is absorbed before adding the next: the rice grains will gradually change colour.

When you've used about half the stock, add the petit pois, and stir through. When the rice is almost cooked but still has a little bite to it – this will take

15–20 minutes depending on the rice – stir in the salmon offcuts, lemon zest and juice and cook for 3 more minutes, stirring occasionally so it doesn't stick. Stir in the cream cheese, if using. Just before serving, scatter the pink peppercorns over the top.

Supper treat

Date and rosewater yogurt pot with almonds (95 cals)

This is another sweet, sleep-enhancing treat with a middle-eastern flavour. Rose water is a subtle flavour: you can buy it in delis or bigger supermarkets, but the strength varies, so experiment with tiny quantities till you get the flavour you like.

The vitamin E in almonds supports the brain and heart, while yogurt and dates are soothing and balancing for the digestive system and blood sugar.

> 3 tablespoons/45g plain or vanilla-flavoured low-fat yogurt, 20–30 cals
> 20g stoned medjool dates, snipped into small pieces, 57cals
> A couple of drops of rosewater (optional)
> A scattering (3g) of toasted flaked almonds, 18 cals

Mix the ingredients together in a small bowl or glass pot, adding the almonds to the top as a garnish.

What to expect this week

- Continued weight loss – sometimes people plateau for a week, but so long as you're eating well but not to extremes the rest of the time, you *will* lose weight.
- More compliments and more energy – and if you're finding ways to improve sleep, even an extra half hour per night will have a big positive effect.

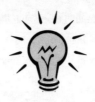

Week 6
DO!

On the menu...

As you celebrate your achievements, it's the ingredients that are the star, prepared with minimum fuss to make the most of their flavours... There's a touch of luxury to mark the end of your plan – and the beginning of the rest of your life! Go on, treat yourself! You deserve it...

Fast day 1

Breakfast
Asparagus royale (106 cals)

When it's in season, asparagus can be really low in price, but it keeps that luxury taste! Here we add smoked salmon for an extra touch of indulgence. If you don't eat fish, serve with a poached egg (see cooking instructions here on page 299)

> 1 small bunch asparagus, 230g, 62 cals
> 20g smoked salmon, 44 cals
>
> OR

1 medium egg, 78 cals
Squeeze of lemon juice
Freshly ground pepper, sea salt

Rinse the asparagus and then cut away the woody stems from the bottoms. (The very thin asparagus spears hardly need any trimming at all.)

Half fill a medium saucepan with water and bring to the boil. Add the asparagus and cook for 4–7 minutes depending on the thickness of the stems. Or you can steam the asparagus in a steamer, or microwave it after rinsing (leave a little water on the stalks to stop them drying out) in a shallow dish for 2–4 minutes, until it's tender but not floppy!

Arrange on a plate with the smoked salmon, season and serve.

Lunch
Melon and Parma ham (110 cals)

A light lunch with a classic combination: the soft, juicy melon and the salty, savoury ham. It doesn't need a dressing, just seasoning, and maybe a few tiny mint leaves as a garnish.

2 slices Parma ham, 62 cals
Around 150g of cantaloupe or honeydew melon, sliced into
    wedges, 48 cals
Salt and pepper
Mint leaves for garnish

Arrange the melon and ham on a plate, season, top with leaves and serve!

Dinner

Halloumi with lemon caper dressing and chilli-roast veg (289 cals)

I love the salty, squeakiness of halloumi, and the intense flavour of the browned bits! The lemon caper dressing has a hint of Greece about it (though use black olives or chillis if you prefer), while the veg add colour and flavour. You can double or triple the portions of veg and keep in the fridge, covered, for a couple of days: it's great with salads or meats or served with crusty bread on a normal day.

100g ripe tomatoes, 20 cals
½ sweet red pepper, seeded and cut into thin strips, 15 cals
½ small fresh chilli, deseeded and chopped finely, 4 cals
100g light halloumi cheese, 240–260 cals
½ teaspoon capers, finely chopped, 1 cal
Juice and zest of ½ a lemon, 9 cals
A few sprigs of fresh thyme or lemon thyme
Freshly ground black pepper

Heat oven to 200°C/400°F/gas mark 6.

Place a piece of foil on a baking tray, add tomatoes, peppers and chilli, curl foil up at the edges to stop juice escaping. Bake for 20 minutes.

Meanwhile, slice the halloumi into thin slices – you want maximum surface area for that lovely browning! Mix the capers and lemon together. Strip the tiny leaves from the thyme stalk using your fingers, and add the leaves to the caper dressing. Keep one sprig whole for serving.

Heat a non-stick frying pan or griddle to a high temperature. Add the halloumi pieces to the pan and cook on one side till the cheese browns and caramelises but doesn't burn. Turn and cook on the other side.

Remove the tomatoes and peppers from the oven, and mix the veg together with a fork, draining off any excess water. Serve the halloumi on top of the veg, with the lemon and caper mix poured on top. Add pepper, but the halloumi will not need any more salt.

Fast day 2

Breakfast

Fresh Alpine strawberries with toasted nut topping (58 cals)

These tiny, pointed strawberries are definitely a luxury, and quite hard to get hold of, but if you see them, snap them up – or grow them in the garden. They are so delicious that they can be served on their own or, as here, with just a few toasted nuts.

Otherwise use normal fresh strawberries – when they're in season (the winter ones often taste more like a rather bitter vegetable to me) – and add a little fat-free Greek yogurt or one of the other topping suggestions.

75g Alpine strawberries (or other strawberries in season), 24 cals
5g toasted almond or hazelnuts, 34 cals

Rinse and pat the strawberries dry, then serve topped with the almonds.

If you're using 'ordinary' strawberries, then these more unusual ideas work well:

- Grind black pepper or crush some pink peppercorns over the top of the strawberries.
- Add a dessertspoon of balsamic vinegar to sliced strawberries and allow to macerate in the fridge for an hour before serving.
- Try rose water or orange flower water sprinkled on top of

the strawberries, followed by a good tablespoon of fat-free Greek yogurt, or half fat crème fraîche. The flower waters vary in strength so try a few drops at first.

Lunch

Mozzarella and fig salad with rocket and balsamic vinegar (235 cals)

More simple ingredients, served *just* so… this makes a seriously pretty plate, too: white, purple, green and yellow. Choose buffalo mozzarella as the flavour and texture are so much better.

½ ball fresh mozzarella, 150–170 cals
20g wild rocket, 5 cals
2 fresh figs, 65 cals
2 teaspoons/10ml balsamic vinegar, 10 cals
Sea salt and black pepper
A small handful of basil leaves, 5 cals
Optional: a scattering of pine nuts (around 10 nuts), 20 cals,
  dry-fried in a pan (watch them as they burn very fast!)

Tear the mozzarella in half and leave the other half in the water (you can use it next day if you keep it submerged and in the fridge).

Lay the rocket on a plate, and slice the figs into quarters through the stalk and arrange them too. Tear the mozzarella half into pieces and lay them on top, pour the balsamic vinegar onto the cheese and salad, season with plenty of salt and pepper. Finally, sprinkle over the pine nuts, if using, and tear over the basil.

The cheese tastes better if served at room temperature so leave it out of the fridge for at least 10 minutes before tucking in!

Dinner

Tarragon poached chicken with grilled artichokes
(230 cals per serving)

Poaching chicken with herbs, wine and baby vegetables is simple but delicious – and this artichoke side dish adds a note of indulgence. But grilling tinned artichokes yourself (look for the ones in brine, not in oil) keeps the costs right down and allows you to control the calories too!

The artichokes make a delicious main for vegetarians if you add goat's cheese and finish under the grill.

I've given amounts for 2 because this is definitely a dish to share!

Tarragon poached chicken

Serves 2

100g trimmed baby carrots, 34 cals

½ bunch of trimmed, baby/small spring onions, roughly chopped, 19 cals

1 celery stick, roughly chopped, 6 cals

OR

50g fennel, roughly sliced, 16 cals

50g broad beans (you can use frozen for this, slip them out of their little greyish 'jackets' before serving), 40 cals

225ml stock made with vegetable or chicken powder/cubes, 12 cals

75ml white wine, 50 cals

1 bay leaf and 3 sprigs of tarragon or thyme

Sea salt and freshly ground pepper

2 small chicken breasts, 240 cals

Grilled artichokes

400g can of artichokes in brine (not oil), drained, 60 cals

For the chicken dish, bring all liquid and flavourings (i.e. everything but the chicken) to the boil in a large saucepan, then turn down to a simmer and place the two chicken breasts in the bottom of the pan. Cover, and cook for 10 minutes. Then turn off the heat and allow the chicken to stay in the liquid for another 20 minutes.

Meanwhile, prepare the artichokes. Drain from the tin and rinse very well to remove the salty taste from the brine. Pat as dry as possible and slice the hearts in half so the inner 'petals' are revealed. You can simply microwave them but I like them griddled, so the edges caramelise. Heat a non-stick griddle to high and then place the artichokes onto the pan (you can use 1-cal spray to prevent sticking). Cook for 2–3 minutes on each side, and allow them to brown before turning over. Season well.

Check the chicken is cooked, then drain the chicken and vegetables, returning the liquid to the heat, bringing it back to the boil and reducing the liquid a little.

Serve the chicken and vegetables plus griddled artichokes, with the poaching sauce on the side.

Tip: For a luxurious-tasting veggie dish for your final day on the programme, top the drained, sliced hearts with 80g mild soft goat's cheese (216 cals), drizzle with ½ teaspoon olive oil (22 cals) and any herbs you fancy, grill till the cheese melts. Serves 2: 149 cals per portion. Serve with a green salad.

What to expect this week

- Elation – and celebration! You should be feeling great as you end the programme. Your clothes will be fitting better, and you'll be feeling much more in control of your eating and – if you've been doing the *5:2 Your Life* plan too – the other things that can make you happy!
- Excited about the next stage? You now have the knowledge and awareness to create your own menu plans, and to eat

342

well on the other days. See 5:2 Flexi-fasting on page 346 – doing it your way for more guidance.

Extra rations

If you're male, or if your Total Daily Energy Expenditure is significantly higher than the average, you can afford to eat a little more than the 500 calories recommended for women on fast days. Most men use 600 as their guideline.

There are two ways to increase the calories – either have a snack during the day, or eat a little more during meals.

I'd personally opt for the second way, because there are some indications that your body benefits more from fasting if you eat less frequently. The easiest way to increase the calories during meals is simply to increase the amount – most of the dishes in the Plan have small portions, and each ingredient is calorie-counted, so you could add an extra egg, 50g more meat or fish, or add a (very small) portion of grated cheese. Alternatively you could cook with fat, rather than 1-cal spray – a single teaspoon of olive oil will add 45 calories to a dish.

See the table over the page for suggestions – as you grow in confidence, try different foods by checking labels. But I advise against adding a biscuit or chocolate bar to your fast days, even if you can find a lower-calorie one; they may trigger cravings or low blood sugar later in the day which can undo your hard work! Also be cautious about fruit if you're eating it as a snack rather than after a meal; berries with natural yogurt, or a kiwi fruit with a small handful of nuts, will help slow down the release of sugars and are a better bet than a banana.

Extra ration	Calories
1 medium egg	78 (plus any fat used to cook)
1 teaspoon oil/butter	45
1 slice bread	55–120 depending on size of loaf
Extra 50g chicken	50–65
100g portion of steamed green veg, e.g. broccoli, green beans	27–30
25g full-fat grated cheddar cheese	100
100g reduced-fat feta-style cheese	90
10g/2 teaspoons seeds, e.g. pumpkin, sunflower	58–65
10 whole almonds	70
50g raspberries with 100g fat-free Greek-style yogurt	75
1 kiwi fruit	42

Emergencies and craving busters

When you're starting out with fasting, there may be times when you really feel like you *need* something to eat. That feeling *will* pass, but it's useful in the early days to have an emergency snack ready, something that contains as few calories as possible, to help you resist the birthday cake being handed round at work, or the family bag of crisps your other half is scoffing on the sofa.

Think about whether any cravings you get tend to be for sweet or for savoury foods, and then choose one or two from the following list to have in your drawer or bag.

If the cravings *do* become overwhelming, you have two choices – if you've only gone over by, say, 100–200 calories, I'd stick with the fast day. If you're invited out, or have something to celebrate, simply fast later in the week.

Snacks	Calories
Miso soup: most sachets of miso soup with tofu or sea vegetables	25–35
10g air popped popcorn (no oil or butter, use herbs or chilli salt for flavour)	31
Olives: 10 pitted green olives	42
Oatcake Plus 2 teaspoons (10g) Philadelphia Light Or 1 teaspoon (5g) peanut butter as a topping	35–50 15 30
Red Mini Babybel Light Babybel	61 40
Sugar-free fruit jelly, per portion	5–15
1 medium plum or peach	40–50
Low-cal hot chocolate, e.g. Options	40–50
1 bite-sized ice-cream bar, e.g. Mini-Milk	30–45
10g 85% dark chocolate	55
10 cherries	40

5:2 Flexi-fasting – doing it your way

One of the best things about intermittent fasting is the flexibility.

We call the approach 5:2, but the fact is, there's no 'magic' about fasting two days a week – you can do one, two, three – or vary the days depending on what your commitments goals are. Welcome to flexi-fasting…

It's perfect if you want a healthier regime, but **hate being told what to eat, when to eat or what to do!** It's also great once you've lost the weight you wanted to lose, and are aiming to maintain.

5:2 is already low on rules – but this version puts you in total control.

How to flexi-fast: 5 steps before starting,

2 guidelines for success

1 **Weigh yourself and calculate your Total Daily Energy Expenditure and personal fast day guideline:** TDEE is an estimate of how many calories you use and so how

many you should consume to maintain your current weight. This is divided by four to get your fast day guideline. You can calculate this via the5-2dietbook.com.

2   **Choose your weight loss target, and how many days per week you want to fast** – weight loss is likely to be more rapid if you fast three days a week, or on alternate days – but it may be harder to sustain. You can vary it – do different days each week, or fast one day this week and three the next. Simply plan the week before and decide what's doable.

3   **Plan your own menus from the recipes in the book** – or to keep it simple, just eat exactly the same every fast day! I know one person who has lost weight by eating two small portions of beans on a slice of wholemeal toast every fast day, and others who choose to consume only fluids. It's your choice.

4   **Check with your doctor before making big changes** (especially if you've decided to eat one meal in the evening, or if you plan a total fast, i.e. to eat nothing at all on your fast day).

5   **Plan to eat normally on your non-fasting days.** To avoid putting on weight, you'll ideally eat to around your TDEE – but you don't have to count calories all the time. You can either be led by your appetite, or try counting one or two 'typical' days to check you're roughly eating the right amount. If you're exceeding your TDEE, then adjust portion sizes or snacking till you're in the right area.

2 ways to monitor your progress

1 **Weigh yourself no more than once a week**, and monitor how it's working for you. If your weight loss isn't quick enough, then increase the number of fast days – but never do more than every other day!

2 When you've reached your goal, **maintain by fasting for one day per week or to suit your own needs.**

My flexi-fasting regime

I reached my target weight after around 5 months of 5:2, though I then adjusted my target downwards by a few pounds – in total I lost 2 stone/28 pounds/13 kilograms.

But as a veteran of so many diets, I knew that losing the weight is only half the battle. Keeping it off can be the hardest part.

Luckily, I felt then – and still feel – very motivated by the health benefits and freedom of intermittent fasting, and so I wanted to stick at it. Many of the 5:2 dieters on our Facebook groups do feel nervous about cutting back to 1 fast day per week, even though for most of us, the approach has helped us to take control of our eating on other days.

I decided to approach it as flexibly as possible. So my new rules are:

1 I fast for one or two days per week, depending on how much I feel I've eaten out or exercised the previous week.

2 I never calorie count on normal days, but I am aware of what my TDEE is and have an awareness too of what that means in terms of my daily diet.

3   No foods are banned, but I am much more 'carb aware' than before and tend to avoid very sugary foods or drinks unless I really fancy them.
4   I never fast on holiday and don't miss out on any treats or special occasions.
5   I tend to eat three or two meals per day, and rarely snack in between meals any more.
6   I never weigh myself after a holiday or a huge dinner – why make yourself feel bad? I know I usually put on a little weight but with 5:2 it'll be gone again soon.

And that's how I'm maintaining my lowest weight for years.

Do I still eat 'too much' sometimes? Yes, some days I eat more than my body needs. Some days I treat myself to a cake to cheer myself up or because I've been offered something too delicious to turn down. But most days I eat in a balanced way.

And I never feel I am missing out.

How *you* flexi-fast will depend on your own needs. You can share your experiences on the *5:2 Diet Book* Facebook group at www.facebook.com/groups/the52diet/

4

TOOLS
FOR YOUR
5:2
LIFE

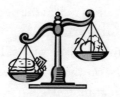

Resources: websites and further reading

The links given in the text are not repeated here – but you will find links to summaries of the main research studies listed in the different chapters. I've used 'bitly' links for the more complicated web addresses, you simply type them into your browser address bar and they go to the sites I've identified.

You can also download a clickable links list for all the links in this book via the website: the5-2dietbook.com – it's *much* easier to use those links than to type in long hyperlinks from this book!

General 5:2 Life and 5:2 Diet Information

For information about 5:2, including the diet and the life plan, visit the5-2dietbook.com.

We have a new Facebook group for this book, facebook.com/groups/52YourLife as well as the original Facebook group, facebook.com/groups/the52diet.

The easiest way to calculate your TDEE is via an online calculator, try the one on the 5-2 website, or fitnessfrog.com/calculators/tdee-calculator.html.

Week 1: Discover

To learn more about the Goal Setting study, go to
    bit.ly/1f786xB.
For information about applying SWOT analysis to personal
    goals, try, bit.ly/MeIdBT.
For more on the Worry O'clock idea, read more at
    bit.ly/1eMpSTA.

Week 2: Connect

For information about the factors involved in happiness, go to the BBC site via this link, bbc.in/1eWPa5X.

For a guide to sprouting seeds, try bitly.com/UaQLK1.

For help with neighbourhood disputes or anti-social behaviour try gov.uk/how-to-resolve-neighbour-disputes – it's a UK government site, but has general advice too.

Abuse and domestic violence:

If you're concerned about abuse or violence in relationships, try the following sources of help:

http://thisisabuse.direct.gov.uk/need-help UK: thisisabuse.direct.gov.uk/need-help.

Australia: http://australia.gov.au/life-events/relationships australia.gov.au/life-events/relationships.

New Zealand: health.govt.nz/your-health/healthy-living/abuse.

Week 3: Simplify

For more on Nicola's shed experiences, type in bit.ly/1h0Lv7i.

Debt advice:

These are good starting points for advice on dealing with debt:

UK: gov.uk/options-for-paying-off-your-debts.

Australia: australia.gov.au/topics/economy-money-and-tax/personal-finance.

New Zealand: cab.org.nz/vat/money/bd/Pages/CreditDebtManagement.aspx.

Week 4: Move

For a review of the science of standing up, read this New York Times article at nyti.ms/1kSKuly – and read more about James Mayo's NEAT work at exm.nr/1hyJAKD.

This article explains the findings about a sedentary life potentially increasing the risk of disability after the age of 60: dailym.ai/1j6WsE4.

This research looks at how being more active affects the brain bit.ly/1iDt0Hv.

Week 5: Relax

Meditation

The headspace site – getsomeheadspace.com – has ten introductory meditations available free: sessions after that are available if you pay a subscription. It's very user-friendly and I like the way mindfulness is explained, plus there's an app so you can listen while you're out and about – very 5:2 friendly!

The UCLA Mindful Awareness Research Center at marc. ucla.edu offers plenty of information, and free guided meditations to download.

Mindfulness for Dummies by Shamash Alidina: I hate the title of this book, but don't judge it by its cover: the tone and explanations are clear and inspiring, with a great CD too. Shamash's personal site also offers a free 3-week mindfulness course by email – see shamashalidina.com.

Week 6: Do!

For career ideas and vacancies, try: gov.uk/jobsearch or jobsite. co.uk in the UK or mycareer.com.au in Australia.

For overall inspiration, but particularly about feeling passionate about what you do in life, it's hard to beat TED.com - a site with inspiring talks about Technology, Entertainment, Design and so much more – it also has free Android and Apple apps to help you widen your horizons wherever you are!

Books

The following books are ones I've enjoyed and found really useful:

The Artist's Way: A Course in Discovering and Recovering Your Creative Self by Julia Cameron. An inspiring book with lots of practical tasks for being more creative in your everyday life. The tone isn't for everyone, though, so do try before you buy. See Julia's own site at juliacameronlive.com.

The Mind Gym: Wake Up Your Mind by the Mind Gym *The Mind Gym* series of books combine research with interesting exercises to try.

My other two 5:2 books, *The 5:2 Diet Book* and *The Ultimate 5:2 Recipe Book* are also available as e-books and print editions.

5:2 Life Planner

A Life Planner can also be downloaded at the5-2dietbook.com.

5:2 YOUR LIFE WEEKLY PLANNER

	WEEK 1	WEEK 2	
5:2 DAY 1 Choose which day/date *Write down:* • activities and challenges you tried • ideas for other activities • how you felt • your own theme			
Notes, thoughts, activities before Day 2			
5:2 DAY 2 Choose which day/date *Write down:* • activities and challenges you tried • ideas for other activities • how you felt • your own theme			
Additional 5:2 activities and plans before the next week			

EK 3	WEEK 4	WEEK 5	WEEK 6

BMI Chart

The Body Mass Index as a measure of whether you're a healthy weight has its limitations, but it is frequently used by doctors and other health professionals, so it's worth knowing where you are on the chart (you can also calculate this at the5-2dietbook. com).

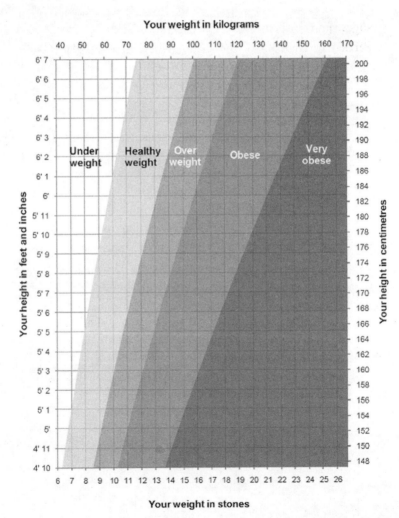

A big thank you...

I want to thank the members of the Facebook group and the 5:2 forum for sharing knowledge and support. It's been an inspiration, from the first days in autumn 2012, when we pooled resources on how to take a basic concept and turn it into a lifestyle, to today when 20,000+ people from all around the world are expanding our knowledge of how making small changes can transform lives, as well as waistlines.

Particular thanks to the team who help me run the community and Facebook groups, and especially to Anita, Boo, Celia, Josie, Linda, Lynda, Megan, Samantha, Skids, Tracey, and Wai. Without you, it'd get very messy indeed! And then there are the girls in the boudoir... you know who you are.

Thanks to Dan Smith for the original sunny cover design which reminds me of a packet of old-school Spangles sweets, and to Amanda Harris, Jillian Young and everyone at Orion for all the hard work turning it into this new, even shinier edition.

This book has grown way beyond my original idea for it, and I am very grateful to the team at LAW for nurturing it, and me, through the process. Special thanks to Elizabeth, Sophie, Araminta and Peta for sweating the big and the small stuff with me, in such a supportive and generous way.

More than ever, I want to thank my family and friends for being there. Much love especially to Mum, Dad, Toni, Geri, Jenny and, of course, to Rich. Every day really is a gift.

Final message from Kate
5:2 *for* Life

Dear Reader,

How's your 5:2 Life right now?

I hope the last six weeks have been fun, and revealing. I've had a fantastic time myself trying out the activities and challenges, and testing *lots* of new recipes.

So what now?

If you're anything like me, then those changes you've made on the two 5:2 days will be having a positive effect on the other days, too. And *5:2 Your Life* is a book you can use again – perhaps as a reboot at certain times of year, or when you want to kick an annoying habit. I tried it again at the start of 2014, and it was just as inspiring as it was the first time. Yes, life, inevitably, gets in the way of our best intentions sometimes, but 5:2 adapts to whatever's going on, so it's easy to get back to good habits when you're ready.

Do check the 5:2 website, too: the5-2dietbook.com – I'm always adding new resources, like my video diary charting my own *5:2 Your Life* journey, and a series of podcasts and downloads to help you, whatever stage you're at.

I'd love to hear your thoughts and experiences – you can contact me via the 5:2 Diet Book website, or my personal website, kate-harrison.com, where you can read about my other books and creative passions. Or share your experiences in our 5:2 Your Life Facebook group, facebook.com/groups/52YourLife – where the stories people are telling inspire me every day.

I hope to see you there!

Kate

Brighton, UK, April 2014

Index

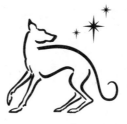

For competitions, author interviews,
pre-publication extracts, news and events,
sign up to the monthly

Orion Books Newsletter

at

www.orionbooks.co.uk

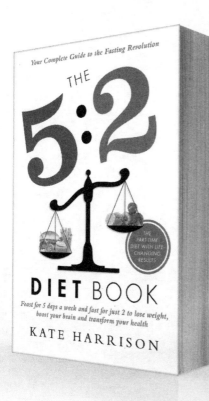
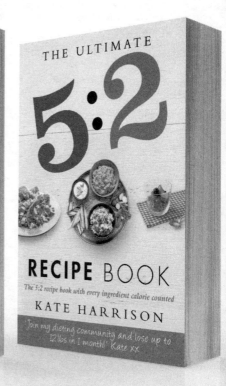